Advance Praise for *Simple Recipes for Joy*

"This beautiful book will transform your life. Sharon Gannon has helped countless people achieve a dramatically new level of health and wellness. Now you can put her wisdom to work as she guides you to using the power of food in ways you may never have imagined. Over many years, our research has established the surprising power of plant-based diets to help people regain their health and vitality. Sharon Gannon brings you everything you need to put that power to work."

— NEAL D. BARNARD, MD, *president, Physicians Committee for Responsible Medicine, and adjunct associate professor of medicine, George Washington University School of Medicine, Washington, DC*

"Sharon Gannon infuses love and spirit into every one of her incredibly delicious dishes; eat her food and feel good in your body and soul!"

— KATHY FRESTON, *New York Times–bestselling author of* Veganist *and* Quantum Wellness

"Sharon is my Guru—I like eating anything she's dishing out. Her teachings on yoga and veganism have positively transformed my life. She is not only an example of someone who walks the talk, but she excels in so many areas: teacher, philosopher, activist, artist, musician and cook, showing us all that through devotion to God one can become a Divine instrument and with God's great love all is possible."

— RUSSELL SIMMONS, *godfather of hip-hop, philanthropist, and author of the* New York Times *bestseller* Super Rich: A Guide to Having It All

"Sharon's food nourishes *and* enlightens. As a longtime devoted fan of her Jivamuktea Café and her yoga teachings, I can't wait to experiment with her alchemy at home. She's finally given up her secrets."

— DARREN ARONOFSKY, *award-winning film director of* Noah, Black Swan, *and* The Wrestler

"All one needs to do is be around Sharon Gannon for mere moments to realize that she's figured out the secret to happiness. Sharon glows with good karma, optimal wellness, and a joyful, blissful life."

—CHLOÉ JO DAVIS, *Eco Spokesmama and GirlieGirlArmy.com founder*

"Super Green Salad, Love Smoothie, Green Machine . . . All enlargements of the soul with the intrinsic beauty of Sharon Gannon, the most impassioned and truthful vegan chef and yogi alive today on Mother Earth."

—JOE SPONZO, *personal chef to Sting and Trudie Styler, and author of* The Lakehouse Cookbook

"Sharon Gannon's beautiful book lies at the untapped intersection of cooking, yoga, and ahimsa practices, demonstrating that preparing and consuming life-giving—rather than life-taking—food is the foundation of a conscious and compassionate life."

—COLLEEN PATRICK-GOUDREAU, *bestselling author of* The Joy of Vegan Baking *and*

The 30-Day Vegan Challenge

"*Simple Recipes for Joy* proves that a compassionate and healthy vegan diet leaves zero to be desired. If you've ever considered leaving animals off your plate, this easy cookbook by one of yoga's masters has a lot to offer. Full of simple yet incredible meat-free recipes, Sharon's recipes are based on wholesome, unprocessed foods that bring us health and vitality. She cooks from the heart, always keeping the well-being of others in mind—both human and animal. She is a tireless voice for the voiceless—and a great cook too!"

—JENNY BROWN, *founder and director of Woodstock Farm Animal Sanctuary and*

author of The Lucky Ones: My Passionate Fight for Farm Animals

"With *Simple Recipes for Joy*, Sharon lets us in on the inner sanctum of her alchemical kitchen. I have had the privilege of sitting at her table since 1979, being personally served by her and eating her delicious, cruelty-free meals—and can attest to the fact that they are filled with nourishment, presented with graciousness and plenty of magic. Her cookbook provides insightful ways to improve our health, the Earth's well-being, and our relationship to our fellow animals, as well as to make positive changes in our diets that will affect the whole world and could possibly save it."

—DR. ANDREW LANGE, ND, *author of* Getting at the Root: Treating the Deepest Source of Disease

"Sharon Gannon does a beautiful job of combining style and substance in life, yoga, and meal preparation. We see that lovely combination on display again with her new cookbook, *Simple Recipes for Joy*. While the book is gorgeous to look at, Sharon's beautifully written introduction points to substantial purpose. The recipes strike a similar balance, teaching us to make delicious food that satiates our senses while nourishing us thoroughly. Sharon has taught countless yogis that the principles of ahisma and asteya, not to harm or steal from others, should guide our food consumption. With these simple recipes, she makes it easy for us to put those principles into action, while enjoying every bite."

—KAREN DAWN, *author of* Thanking the Monkey

"Buying a vegan cookbook is usually an expression of interest. Buying this one is a declaration. The activism known as peace springs from your plate—and thanks to Sharon Gannon, it's a delectable beginning."

—KEVIN ARCHER, *author of* In Lieu of Heaven

Simple Recipes for Joy

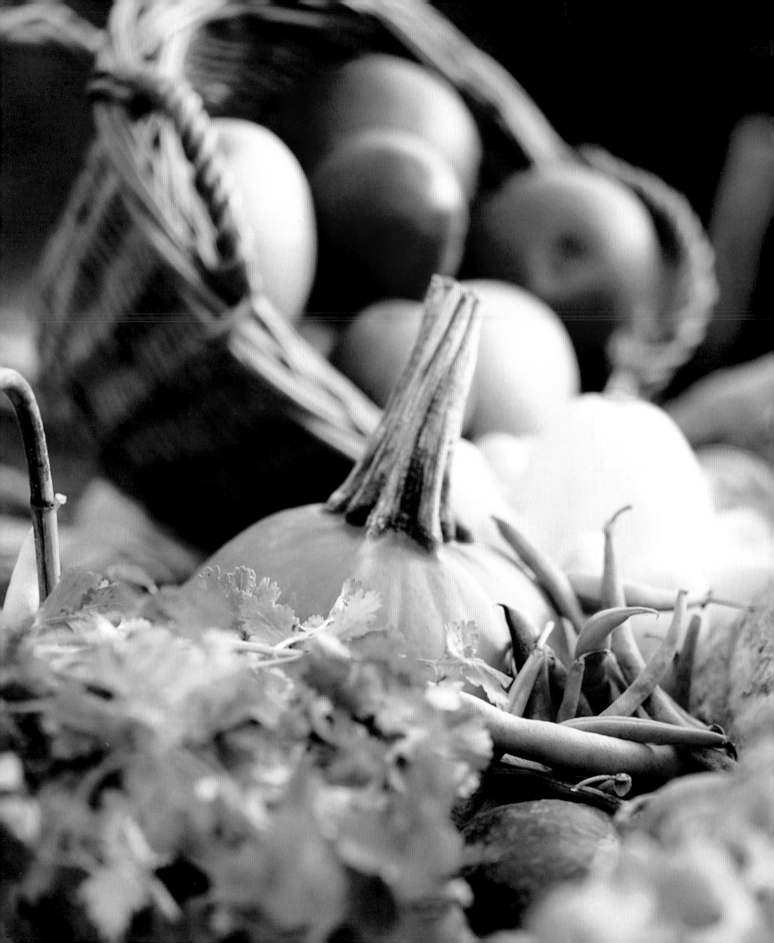

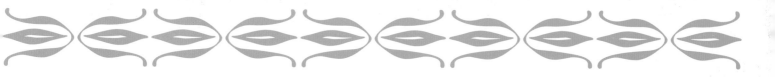

Simple Recipes
for Joy

More Than 200 Delicious
Vegan Recipes

SHARON GANNON

FOREWORD BY KRIS CARR

AVERY · an imprint of Penguin Random House · New York

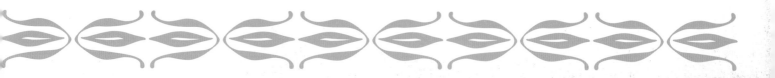

an imprint of Penguin Random House LLC
375 Hudson Street
New York, New York 10014

First trade paperback edition 2016
Copyright © 2014 by Sharon Gannon
Photographs on pages ix, 52, 100, 113, 224, 230, 236, 260, 267, 280 © 2014 by Jessica Sjöö
Photographs on pages 19 and 267 © 2014 by David Life
Photograph on page 4 © 2014 by Bill Miles
All other photographs © 2014 by Guzman

Most Avery books are available at special quantity discounts for bulk purchase for sales promotions, premiums, fund-raising, and educational needs. Special books or book excerpts also can be created to fit specific needs. For details, write SpecialMarkets@penguinrandomhouse.com.

The Library of Congress has catalogued the hardcover edition as follows:

Gannon, Sharon.
Simple recipes for joy : more than 200 delicious vegan recipes / Sharon Gannon ; foreword by Kris Carr.
p.   cm.
ISBN 978-1-58333-559-8
1. Vegan cooking.   I. Title.
TX837.G288   2014   2014009063
641.5'636—dc23

ISBN 978-1-58333-588-8 (paperback)

Printed in the United States of America
1 3 5 7 9 10 8 6 4 2

Printed on recycled paper

Book design by Gretchen Achilles

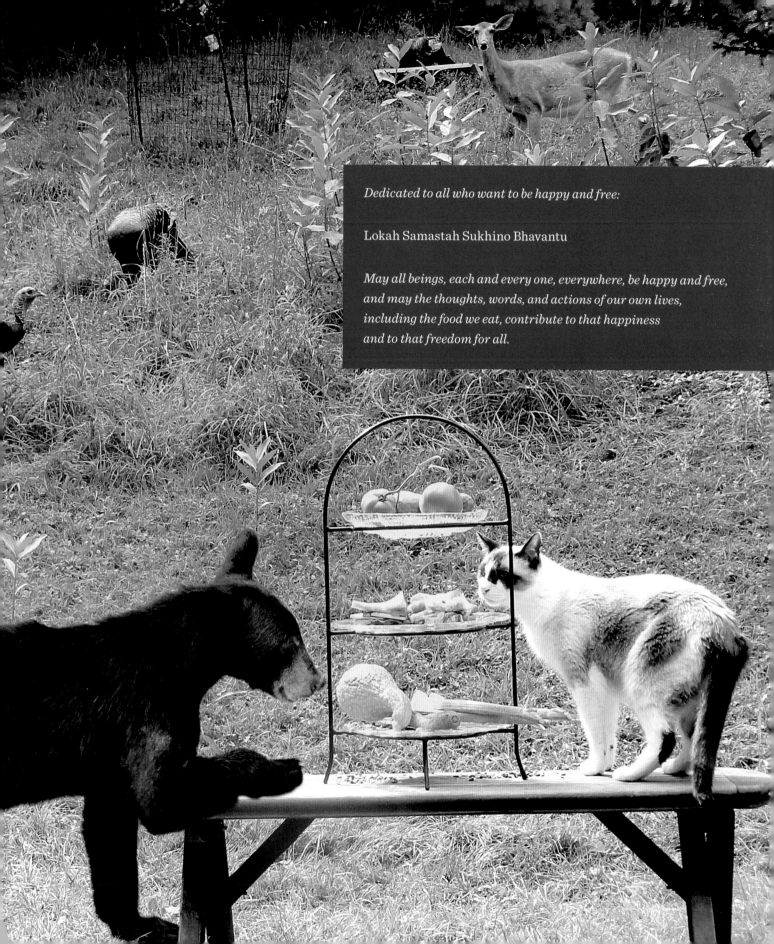

Dedicated to all who want to be happy and free:

Lokah Samastah Sukhino Bhavantu

*May all beings, each and every one, everywhere, be happy and free,
and may the thoughts, words, and actions of our own lives,
including the food we eat, contribute to that happiness
and to that freedom for all.*

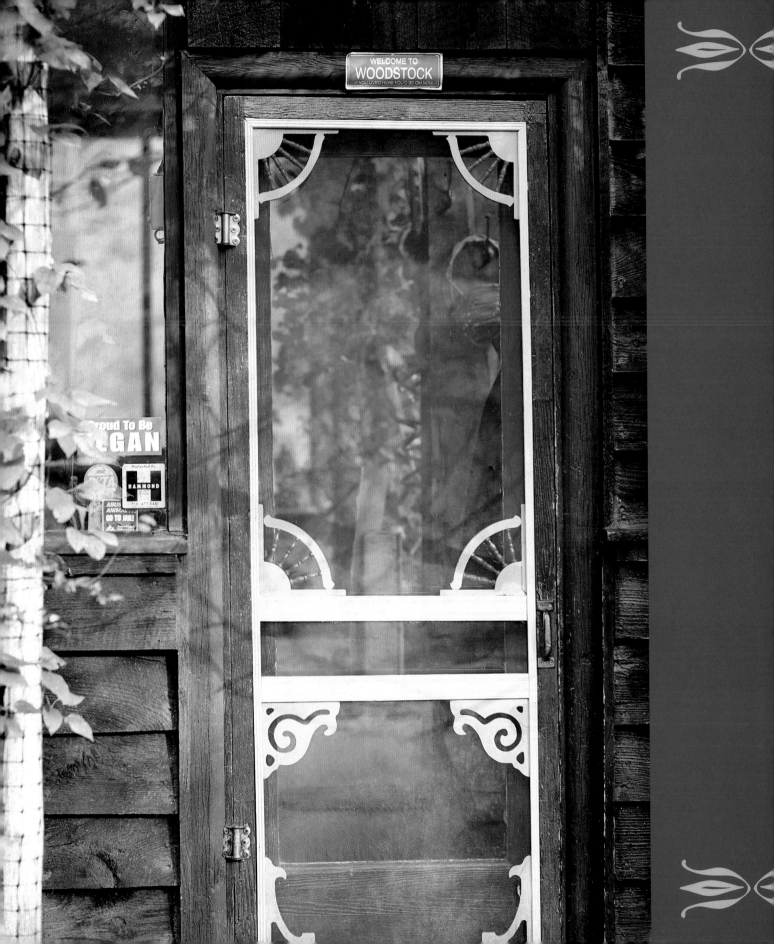

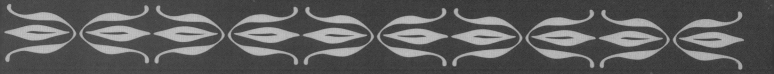

Contents

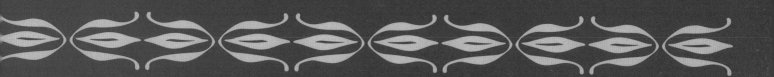

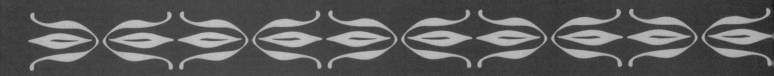

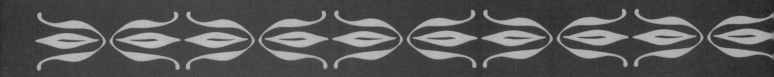

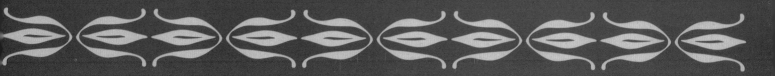

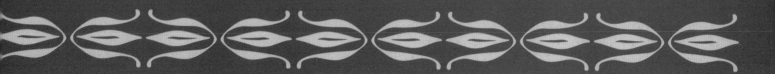

Simple Recipes for Joy

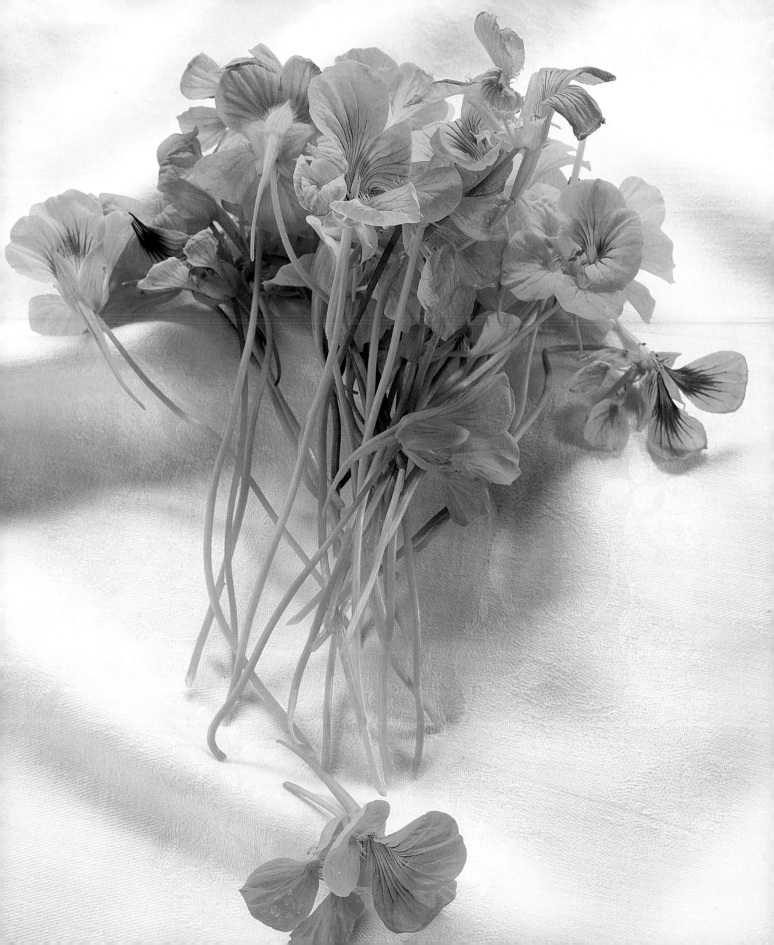

Foreword

Sharon Gannon's latest book has the power to change your life; it may even save it. This is a pretty bold statement. After all, you're holding only a cookbook, right? Wrong. Trust me, this statement is spot-on accurate. How do I know? Because Sharon's teachings are part of the reason I'm alive. And her recipes are more than a healthy meal; they are the foundation of what's known as functional, holistic medicine. You see, the doctor of the future is you. You know exactly what your body needs to thrive and by quieting your mind, dumping your addictions, and listening to your gut wisdom, you too will learn how to use food to transform your life.

Food literally has the power to heal and the power to poison. In my journey as a cancer patient, I've come to understand that health is not an absence of disease; it is a presence of vitality, sustainable energy, and joy. Health is our birthright. And yet so many of us have forgotten. We believe that our genes determine our fate and that we have no control over our lives. This couldn't be further from the truth. The genes you were born with are not your destiny. Your daily food choices (along with your lifestyle and environment) affect your genetic future. That's right: what you eat today can literally have an impact on your DNA. Which is precisely why many people who follow the Standard American Diet (SAD) are sick, overweight, tired, and in a state of total dis-ease.

The SAD way of living, filled with acidic animal products that are high in saturated fat, cholesterol, and cancer-causing carcinogens, processed foods, and refined sugar, strips our bodies of minerals and creates oxidative stress and inflammation. In fact, inflammation is the root cause of most chronic diseases. Inflammation is like being on fire on the inside, and this fire (or stress) comes from what we eat, drink, and think. In the case of animal products, the more we consume, the more inflamed and sicker we become.

It's actually pretty ironic. We torture and slaughter billions of sentient beings each year because we erroneously believe that we need to eat their bodies for proper nourishment. "Milk, it does a body good," right? "Beef, it's what's for dinner." These messages have been strategically carved into our brains. Yet, this so-called nourishment often sends us to the grave earlier than necessary. It's such a waste.

And who propagates these myths? The food industry. With billions of advertising dollars at their disposal, we are led to believe that meat, dairy, eggs, fish, poultry, processed foods, sugary snacks, and sodas are good for us. Because there is little regulation, we are incredibly vulnerable and often confused. As a result we blindly consume the foods that lead to heart disease, stroke, cancer, diabetes, obesity, hypertension, osteoporosis, arthritis, and so on. Let's pause for a moment and follow the money trail. If plant-based foods are so good for us, then why can they sometimes be more expensive? Special interests do not favor broccoli. The fast-food burger is cheap because of government subsidies. And yet, calorie per calorie, there is more nourishment (vitamins, minerals, fiber, phytonutrients, antioxidants, and even protein!) in broccoli than in steak. So is cheap food a wise investment? No way. And once you learn how to shop wisely, you'll see that a plant-based diet can fit into any budget.

It's that simple, and yet we're so confused. I know I certainly was. I was a hard-core omnivore and a junk-food junkie for many years. But on February 14, 2003, everything changed. Happy Valentine's Day, you have cancer—a rare stage-IV disease with no treatment (no chemo, radiation, or surgery) and no cure. I was devastated. The first doctor I consulted suggested a triple organ transplant to remove and replace my liver and both of my lungs. Because these organs were riddled with malignant tumors, he thought it was my only hope. The second doctor suggested another radical treatment (that wouldn't cure me) and gave me just ten years to live. I was only thirty-one years old. In an instant, I thought my life was over. I had no idea it was just getting started. I finally found an open-minded oncologist who helped me decide upon a radical approach. Watch and wait. Do nothing. Since the disease could be slow-moving, maybe I had time.

As it turns out, I did have time, and I decided to use it wisely. Next stop, Whole Foods, my pharmacy. How did I know to go to Whole Foods and stock up on plant-powered medicine? Sharon Gannon.

I started practicing Jivamukti yoga in 1991. At the time I was a young dancer, actress, and bartender with lots of injuries and "isms." Jivamukti quickly became my church. It was a place I could go to take care of my temple and find my way home. I had never heard of veganism before studying with Sharon. I barely knew how to sit still, let alone make a bowl of quinoa! But slowly I began to listen.

When the diagnosis came, I listened at the deepest level imaginable. Here's what I heard: "Practice yoga, learn how to take care of yourself, reduce your stress load, calm your mind, sleep, and most important—change what's on your plate." Influenced by Sharon's teachings of ahimsa (nonviolence), I decided to practice kindness and compassion toward all beings, including myself. The first step was to remove stimulants like caffeine, alcohol, and sugar, all processed foods, and all animal products from my diet. After the initial detox period, I was astonished by how great I felt. For the next eight years, I researched the diets and lifestyles that were known to increase immunity, strength, and longevity. Guess what? They were all plant-based.

At this point, you may be questioning why your doctor hasn't told you any of this information, or worse, you may wonder why he or she won't validate these findings. The truth is that doctors don't study nutrition in medical school. Therefore it's our job to teach ourselves.

For nearly a decade now, I have lived a happy, healthy, and stable life in the face of a deadly disease. I still have cancer but it doesn't have me. The diagnosis that once terrified me continues to lie dormant. Thanks to my diet and lifestyle, I'm in terrific overall health and have boundless energy, peace, and strength.

In the process of learning about the power of foods, I've had the privilege to share these principles with thousands of people from around the world, many of whom have been able to fully restore their health naturally without drugs, surgeries, or complicated and costly medical procedures. Like Sharon, I can't think of a better way to spend my life than in the service of others. Because once we learn this information, we must pay it forward by spreading this lifesaving message to our families and friends.

As a nation we are getting sicker and fatter. Every day, fifteen hundred people die of cancer. Every minute a person in the United States dies of heart disease. Two-thirds of adults are overweight or obese. And diabetes is growing at an alarming rate. Young people are being diagnosed with diseases common to their grandparents, and many researchers believe that the next generation will be the first to die before their parents. Health care costs are ballooning out of control, yet most of the money goes toward treating diseases that are preventable with proper plant-based nutrition. It's easy to conclude that the leading cause of death in this country is not disease, it's an unhealthy diet.

At the same time, our precious environment urgently cries out for help. According to the United Nations, "livestock are responsible for 18 percent of greenhouse gas emissions, a bigger share than that of transport. Livestock now use more than 30 percent of the Earth's entire land surface. As forests are cleared to create new pastures, it is a major driver of deforestation, especially in Latin America, where 70 percent of former forests have been turned over to grazing. The livestock business is also among the most damaging sectors to the Earth's increasingly scarce water resources, contributing among other things to water pollution from animal wastes, antibiotics and hormones, chemicals from tanneries, fertilizers and the pesticides used to spray feed crops."

Now, this all may seem depressing at first, but it's also thoroughly empowering if you're willing to do something. But know this: We can't wait for change. We must *be* the change. You can change the world from your kitchen. You can lead a peaceful plant-based protest, but only if you're willing to buck the broken system and take a compassionate stand for yourself, the animal beings, and the precious world around you.

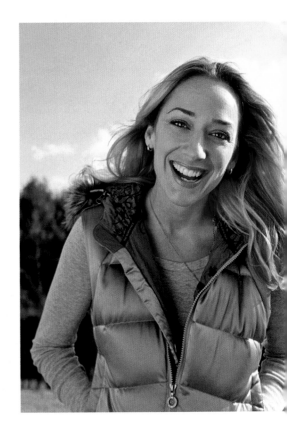

Take it from me: prevention is the only lasting cure. No matter what your circumstance, actively participating in your health, spiritual wealth, and happiness is a revolutionary act. Join the revolution today. Read this book, try the delicious recipes, and tell everyone you know to do the same. Listen to Sharon. She is a true visionary, a pioneer, and a compassionate mother to many beings. I'm so grateful to her for teaching me how to heal. Now she will teach you.

Peace, love, and veggies,

KRIS CARR, bestselling author of *Crazy Sexy Diet* and *Crazy Sexy Cancer Tips*

Introduction

It's a Tuesday afternoon in New York City, and Union Square is as hectic and bustling as ever. People pass our Broadway entrance looking harried, barking into cell phones, lugging overstuffed briefcases, tugging toddlers' hands. But inside the Jivamukti Yoga School, the creases of worry on the people's faces fade away. After a peaceful yoga class, many of them step into Jivamuktea Café for a Chakra Rainbow Smoothie (pages 298–300), a Burrito Verdura (page 250), or some Spirulina Millet (page 180). They linger to talk—laughing quietly, reading, or simply sitting—at home in the tranquillity and joy that abounds in this place.

Serving them, I am filled with gladness. I learned long ago that if I wanted to find enlightenment, cooking was the first step, and that if I was in search of joy, there was no better way to reach it than by providing for others. Yogis, who live by the nonviolent yogic principle of ahimsa, naturally gravitate toward the all-vegan, cruelty-free menu at Jivamuktea Café; and the simple peace and joy that fills them as they sit down to eat infuses the entire room with happiness.

As a child, I asked my mother, "If killing is wrong, isn't it wrong to eat animals?" My mother replied, "It is okay, because they are raised for that." Like most people, she felt that eating enslaved animals was normal and acceptable. Due to what they eat, many human beings on the planet today consciously or unconsciously cause tremendous harm to themselves, to the environment, and to billions of animals.

For most, what they eat is influenced by unconscious habits, ignorance, and mass media advertising rather than common sense, kindness, or joy. I have been reminded time and time again of the power of the printed word. Cookbooks, food critics, and celebrities can have a huge influence on what people choose to eat and whether or not restaurants stay open. The animal-user industries of course are well aware of this and pay a lot of money to get celebrities to endorse their products. Remember the milk mustache? And it's worked; most of us have become so *civilized* that we can't think for ourselves. Common sense is not so common. We

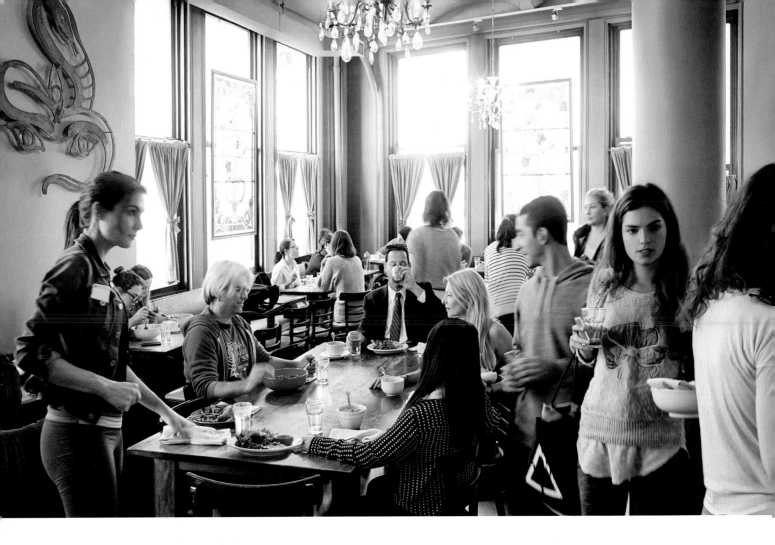

have relinquished our innate sense and sensibilities, giving them over to the advertising agencies and food critics to manipulate our appetites.

In fact, we too often have no appetite outside of what we have become programmed to crave. As we have dissociated ourselves from nature, we have also become disconnected from the natural intelligence of the body. We can no longer feel what our bodies really need; we live in our heads, and our heads have been thoroughly programmed by our culture. We have allowed our own bodies to become so polluted by and addicted to junk food, tainted animal flesh, and milk products that we cannot even tell anymore when we are consuming something poisonous and injurious to our health. We have allowed "Food Inc."—corporations and the animal-user industries, which have in many cases become more powerful than governments—to decide what's available and affordable to eat. In America, Froot

Loops (a highly processed, high-fructose, genetically modified, corn-based breakfast cereal) is cheaper to buy per serving than a piece of real organic fruit! Everything that is good for us and good for the environment has been stigmatized with the label *alternative*, while foods that are harmful to our health and the health of the environment are called *normal* or *standard*, and that is sad.

Some people may argue that they have a right to eat meat and dairy products, saying that it is nobody's business what they do. When a person defends their right to eat meat and dairy products, they are failing to realize the devastating impact that such a diet has upon the environment and all of the life on this planet. It is fair to assume that most meat eaters are not eating meat because they want to cause harm to an animal or the environment; it is most likely more a matter of not thinking further than what appeals to their appetite at the moment. I think meat eaters generally view veganism as no more than a dietary preference, similar to preferring chocolate over vanilla, not realizing the life-and-death seriousness of the issue. When you are a meat eater, you generally don't bring consciousness to your food choices. Of course some do, like people who eat kosher or halal food, or Catholics who abstain from meat on Fridays, or others with food allergies to gluten, peanuts, etc. But nevertheless, out of the worldwide human population of seven billion, very few meat eaters bring any significant level of awareness to the food on their plates. For the vast majority of people, food choices are a matter of habit, convenience, and personal preference rather than ethical considerations. They will just eat whatever is being served, whatever appeals to them on the menu, as the flight attendant asks, "Chicken or beef?"

When we become aware of the atrocities that are being committed against defenseless animals, many of us feel saddened and even overwhelmed. We feel helpless to do something about it all. Confronting or even discussing the issue with our family and friends can feel overwhelming, not to mention the helplessness we may feel against the forces of government or multinational corporations. How could any of us make a difference in a world where the majority of human beings feel it is not only normal and okay to eat animals but it is our God-given right as the dominant species to exploit the weak?

It is a fact that our consumption of meat, eggs, and dairy is excessive, yet our culture is founded upon the excessive enslaving and exploiting of animals for food. This way of life started around ten thousand years ago, when human beings began to domesticate animals and exploit them for material gain as part of the shift from a nomadic lifestyle to a more sedentary one.[1] So the good news is that eating animals and animal products is not hardwired into us—it is cultural, something we have learned. Behaviors and habits that are learned can be unlearned, if exposed to enlightening education.

Our relationship to food is fundamental to our existence. Who can deny the importance that food plays in our lives? It sustains us physically, emotionally, and even spiritually, because without a physical body the spirit has no vehicle through which to experience life. Eating is the most essential way that we as human beings relate to the Earth—to nature. Eating is also the most essential way that we relate to each other. The most basic relationship in the human/animal world is between a parent and child. The primal relationship between a mother and her baby is based on the mother providing food for her dependent baby by means of her own breast milk. Without mother's milk, most newborn infant mammals would die. Meals shared with family and friends play a valuable role in the development of social ties. Whole societies are built upon food—the planting, harvesting, storing, trading or selling, and preparation of food.

For many of us who consume meat and dairy products, food is the only way that we relate to animals. Peter Singer, author of the groundbreaking book *Animal Liberation* (first published in 1975), has so aptly observed, "Most of us relate to animals three times a day when we sit down to eat them." "That's a terrible way to define a relationship," adds Ingrid Newkirk, founder of PETA.

My own personal relationship with food has taken me into various worlds of eating and not eating. As a child, I endured times of starvation due to financial difficulties, and I learned the power that imagination plays in regard to food. My brother, sister, and I would take the condiments and spices out of a pretty much bare cupboard, sprinkle salt and pepper into our palms, and "tongue taste." As we licked up the salt and pepper we would "savor," imagining we were eating a baked potato. A bit of cinnamon would transport us into a world filled with pumpkin pie or French toast. The interesting thing was that after such a "virtual meal," we didn't feel so hungry. As a young woman, I was anorexic for seven years due to severe emotional trauma. During that time, I became very sensitive and could feel the minute effects of a sip of water or a crumb of bread in my body. Experiences like these have taught me how powerful our thoughts can be in regard to food.

Since immersing myself in the practices of yoga, I have become aware of how offering food to God before eating it transforms the experience of eating into a sacred act.

Ironically, after dropping out of college during my first year—due to a nervous breakdown brought on by lack of food coupled with the stress of living with my boyfriend, who was starving himself to obtain a draft deferment from the Vietnam War—I went into the restaurant business. Partnering with my boyfriend and another friend, the three of us opened our own restaurant in Seattle in 1971. Hunger is what motivated us. We called the restaurant You Are What You Eat. None of us knew very much about cooking or running a business, but we did know that we were hungry.

Hunger can be a very passionate motivator, and passion tends to attract attention. Our little restaurant became

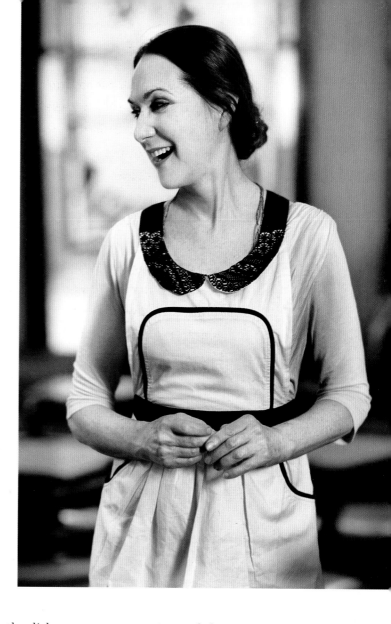

an overnight success. The food was tasty, the dishes were very creative, and the portions a bit too generous for the prices we charged. The decor was whimsical and swinging—one table actually sported a swing seat, a wooden plank hanging by two chains mounted in the ceiling. Instead of a conventional chair, a customer could dine while swaying in a swing. Milton Katims, the then conductor of the Seattle Symphony, was a regular customer and was outspoken with his enthusiasm for my cooking, especially the borscht, about which he would remark, "Sharon, this is as good as my Russian grandmother's! With no beef stock, how do you do it?"

At the time there were no vegetarian restaurants in Seattle and items on our menu such as alfalfa sprouts, soy nuts, and avocado sandwiches were hard to find.

Even though there was a heavy emphasis on vegetarian dishes at You Are What You Eat, it wasn't a vegetarian restaurant. I was not a vegan at the time, and my two partners were voracious omnivores. We were hippies, and, like most of our contemporaries, we had been influenced by the vegetarianism of the Beatles and the *Farm Vegetarian Cookbook*, but also, unfortunately, the non-vegetarianism of Arlo Guthrie's *Alice's Restaurant Cookbook*. You Are What You Eat stayed open for a little less than a year but had to close when the landlord sold the property to an oil company to build a gas station. After we closed the restaurant, I focused on developing myself as an artist for the next decade or so.

My life changed forever in 1982, when I saw a British documentary film titled simply *The Animals Film*. The film exposed many of the cruel and exploitive ways that human beings treat animals—all of which are considered quite normal in our culture. It explored the use of animals as entertainment, food, providers of clothing, and subjects in scientific and military experiments.

I had been an on-again, off-again vegetarian before the film, but shortly afterward I became a vegan and shortly after that a yoga teacher. I incorporated veganism and animal rights in all the work I did as my way of taking direct action against the cruelty inflicted upon other animals by us, human beings. And I started to educate myself about the damage done by the Standard American Diet.

According to U.S. Department of Agriculture statistics, in the United States 10 billion land animals are slaughtered every year for food, and approximately 53 billion sea creatures are slaughtered every year worldwide for American consumption—that's 63 billion individual beings killed![2] The number is staggering when you consider that there are only 7 billion human beings on the entire planet— and we're talking here just about the number of animals killed by human beings in only *one* country in *one* year.

Then there is the water issue. Fresh, clean drinking water is rapidly becoming a scarce commodity. One in every seven people in the world today does not have access to clean water.[3] Most of the water that is consumed is used to raise animals for food.[4] It takes 2,400 gallons of water to produce a pound of meat, but only twenty-five gallons to produce a pound of wheat. A vegan diet requires three hundred gallons of water per day;[5] a meat-eating diet requires more than 4,000 gallons of water per day.[6] Raising animals for food causes more water pollution than any other industry.[7] Much of the waste from farms, which contains high levels of toxic chemicals from pesticides, herbicides, antibiotics, hormones, and other pharmaceuticals, flows into and contaminates streams, groundwater, rivers, and oceans.

As for the benefits of going vegan: a vegan diet has been proven to reverse and prevent heart disease[8] and cancer,[9] and there is growing evidence that it can successfully treat diabetes.[10] Vegans on average live longer than meat eaters and they weigh less.[11] (Meat and dairy consumption makes you fat and can even contribute to erectile dysfunction in men.[12]) Perhaps most important, by eating a plant-based diet, you contribute to more joy in the world and in yourself.

In 1983, I moved to New York City to further the career as a musician/artist that I had begun in Seattle after You Are What You Eat closed. To support myself, I worked as a cook and as a waitress in David Life's Life Café. Because of the awareness I had developed about the impact of meat-eating on our bodies, other animals, and the environment, I am proud to say that I influenced the Life Café to become the first restaurant in New York City to offer a soy milk cappuccino and other vegan dishes. Though the Life Café did come to offer many vegetarian and vegan options, it was not strictly a vegetarian restaurant.

The Life Café provided David with his main source of income, but when he and I started to teach more and more yoga classes, the meat on the café menu started to bother him. He found it more and more difficult to justify serving hamburgers and omelets. Then John Robbins's book Diet for a New America came out in 1987. David read the book, and after he was done he read it again. After the second reading, he put the book down, walked over to the Life Café, told his partner that he was finished and she could have his percentage of the business; he didn't want a monetary settlement. She asked him, "What will you do now? How will you support yourself?" And he answered, "I'm not sure of that, but I am sure of one thing, and that's that I'm not going to make my living by causing the death of animals."

David and I had faith that by teaching yoga in a way that was aligned with the ethical precepts, which included ahimsa—a practice that attempts to minimize the harm one causes—the universe would guide and take care of our needs. Fortune smiles on the brave, they say, and so it came to pass that more and more people came knocking on our door wanting yoga classes. The heavy animal rights and vegan message in the classes we taught didn't seem to put them off, and our school quickly became very popular and outgrew three spaces.

Veganism and yoga are natural partners. The Sanskrit word *yoga* means "to link, to connect," and that implies relationship. Asana, which is perhaps the most well-known of the many yogic practices, to many just means physical exercises like standing on your head or back bending. But the term *asana* actually means how one connects or relates to the Earth. In the *Yoga Sutra*, Patanjali says that our relationship to the Earth (*asana*) should be steady (*sthira*) and joyful (*sukham*), if we desire yoga—enlightenment, ultimate happiness, freedom from suffering. A yogi is someone who strives to live harmoniously with the Earth and all beings.

A yogic lifestyle is radical because it challenges the very root of our present culture—a culture economically based on enslaving, exploiting, and eating animals. What sets the yogi apart from most normal people today is that a yogi wants liberation, or *moksha*. A yogi realizes that how we treat others will determine how others treat us, how others treat us will determine how we see ourselves, and how we see ourselves will determine who we are.

Yoga teaches that whatever we want in life we can have if we are willing to provide it for others. So if yogis want to be free, they understand that to deprive others of freedom will ultimately not benefit their project—to be free themselves. Following that logic, yogis abhor slavery and examine their own lives to find ways that they themselves might be condoning slavery and then eradicate those ways of acting. The fact is that animals who are raised for food are slaves. Making kind choices when it comes to the food we eat is one of the most basic ways to begin to ensure our own happiness and freedom. The cause for our own happiness, health, and freedom lies in how happy and free we can make the lives of others. The definition of *others* includes other animals.

In 2006 we opened the Jivamukti Yoga School at 841 Broadway, off Fourteenth Street, in New York City and with it, the elegant, seventy-seat Jivamuktea Café, serving organic teas as well as organic vegan food seven days a week. Our statement of purpose for our café and for our school is the same: *Jivamukti Yoga is a path to enlightenment through compassion for all beings. Jivamukti is a Sanskrit word that means to live liberated in joyful, musical harmony with the Earth. The Earth does not belong to us—we belong to the Earth. Let us celebrate our connection to life by not enslaving animals and exploiting the Earth, and attain freedom and*

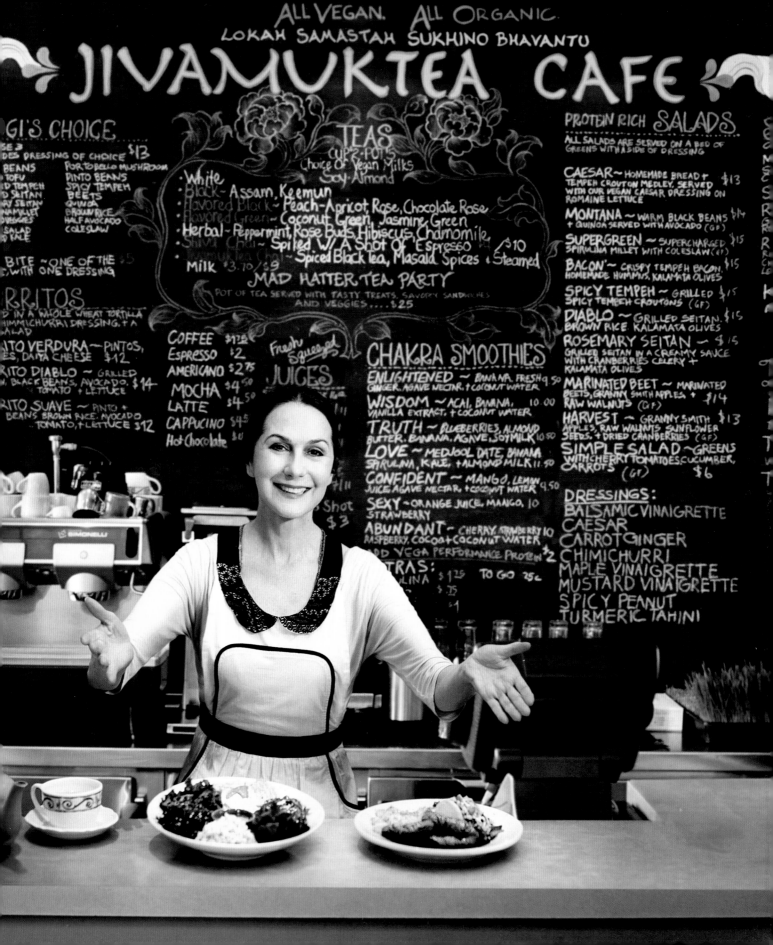

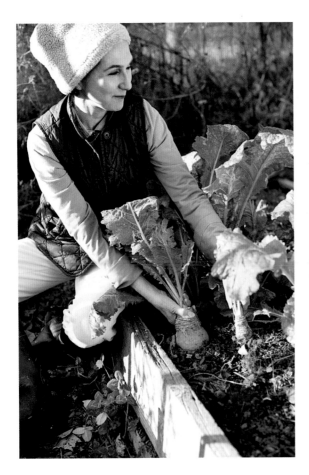
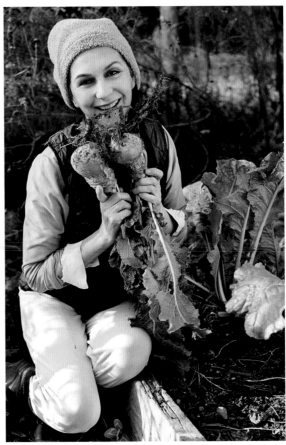

happiness for ourselves in the process. For surely, the best way to uplift our own lives is to do all we can to uplift the lives of others. Go vegan!

I asked my first spiritual teacher, the alchemist Randy Hall, "How do I become enlightened?," and he responded, "First, learn how to cook, clean, and garden." I started to put that into practice when I became vegan, and I began to share it with others on a grand scale with Jivamuktea Café, creating a menu of vegan dishes that are delicious and designed to bring peace and joy to the chef, the staff, the diners, the animals, and the planet.

Preparing and cooking food is an alchemical practice: deftly combining varied ingredients and subjecting them to the elements of water, fire, and air in just the right proportions and with just the right timing and appropriate spells—consisting of good mental intentions, with no gossip or small talk in the kitchen—to manifest a delicious meal that satisfies both body and soul. Food prepared in this way can even produce a magical shift in perception of oneself and others, yielding hope and encouragement to move forward through life!

So what exactly does it mean to be vegan? To eat a vegan diet means that you eat a 100 percent plant-based diet: you eat vegetables, you don't eat any animal products, and you do this for ethical reasons—out of compassion for the animals and the Earth as well as respect for yourself and for life itself. Some people may say they are vegetarians but still eat milk products, eggs, and fish. Vegans do not eat dairy products, eggs, honey, or fish because these are not vegetables and eating them causes great harm. Some clarification about what constitutes animal products: *animal products* pertains to the muscles, flesh, fat, organs, milk, fluids, blood, saliva, eggs, unborn fetuses, and infants that come from the body of an animal. The term *animal* refers to any living being, which includes all species of mammals, birds, fish, amphibians, reptiles, and insects.

In other words, a vegan would not eat any part of or any substance produced by a cow, which includes their milk, blood, testicles, hooves (gelatin), brains, liver, kidney, or intestines, or any part of or any substance produced by a pig, sheep, goat, chicken, turkey, duck, goose, fish, frog, snake, or bee (honey). Nor would a vegan refer to any fellow Earthling by using derogatory terms such as *beef, pork, mutton,* or *poultry*—all of which indicate the categorizing of a living being according to his or her exploitable, edible resources.

Many vegans extend their ethics to include not just what they eat but everything they consume: food, clothing, furnishings, medicine, and entertainment, to name a few. Vegans do not view animals as existing to be used by human beings. A

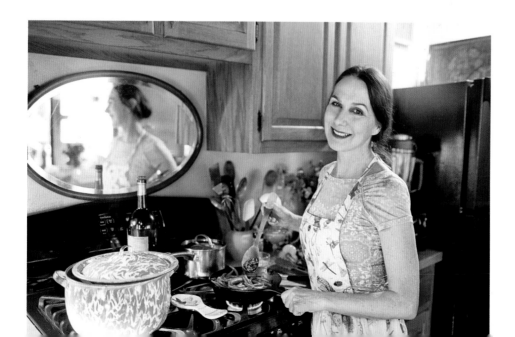

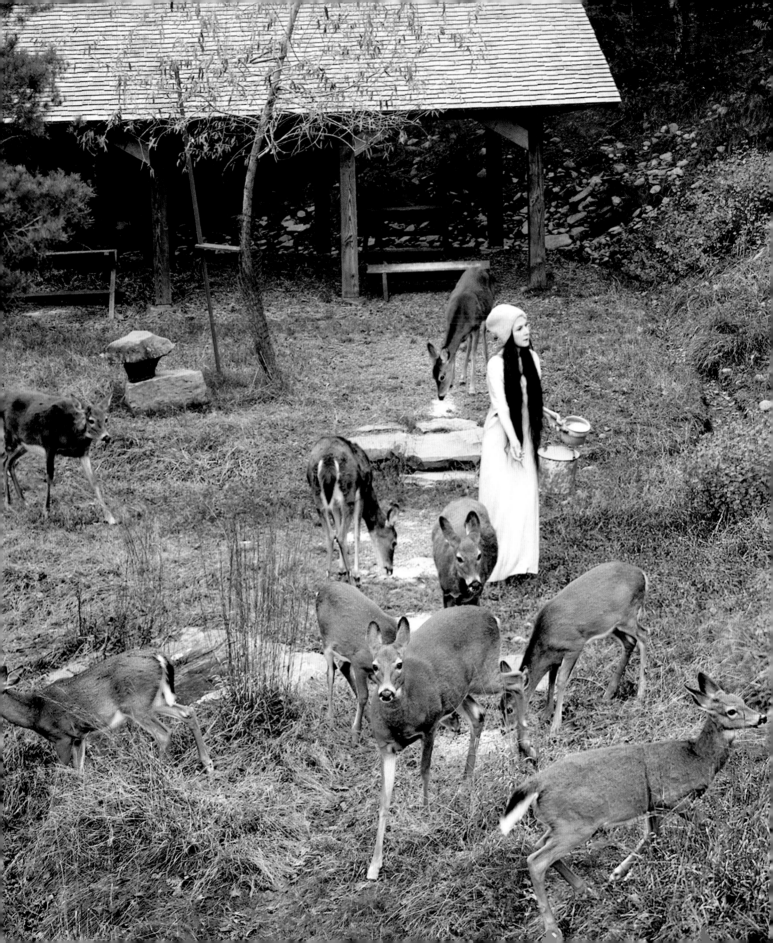

vegan is an abolitionist who abhors slavery. Most humans believe that slavery and concentration camps are a shameful thing of the past. But the fact is that billions of animal beings are cruelly confined in today's concentration camps: the modern industrial factory farms—CAFOs (confined animal feeding operations). And even animals who are raised for food on small family-owned farms and on fish farms are slaves—they are confined to serve the interests of their "owners" with no rights to live full, happy lives true to their nature. A person who eats enslaved animals is not only condoning slavery but sustaining it as the foundation of our global economy. People who adopt a vegan diet solely for health reasons may not be motivated by a desire to see the end of slavery and exploitation of animals, but their dietary choices further those ends just the same.

In truth, the Standard American Diet (SAD) is sad because it is not healthy for humans, animals, or the environment. A plant-based, vegan diet is the healthiest diet for human beings. A vegan's negative impact upon the environment is substantially lower than a meat eater's, and a vegan diet is obviously kinder to animals. When you have a simple choice to be kind or cruel, why not choose to be kind and, by doing so, contribute to raising the level of joy and happiness in the world?

We are in the midst of a global crisis. The living world is dying in our time. I hope that the book you hold in your hands will help to provide you with the means to begin to heal the global crisis, saving this planet from destruction. To be a joyful vegan in the world today is to become involved in the most radical, positive, political revolution ever. A fork can be a weapon of mass destruction or an instrument of peace. Everything a vegan eats or consumes reflects a choice that takes into account the well-being of others rather than just ourselves—and that *is* a big difference. Each one of us can make a huge difference by choosing not to eat animals. By choosing kindness over cruelty, we contribute to the sustainability of our planet Earth and can even change the destiny of our species and all the species on Earth.

Simply put, this is a book of formulas, complete with how-to instructions, suggestions, and advice, which, if followed with a cheerful heart and sense of adventure, could result in the most delightful culinary experiences manifesting on your dinner table. But don't worry—use these recipes as guidelines; feel free to improvise, as seasoned cooks do. Most of the recipes for the dishes, drinks, and desserts that are served in Jivamuktea Café are contained in this book, plus a whole lot more. Many of the photos come from the café, and the rest come from my home

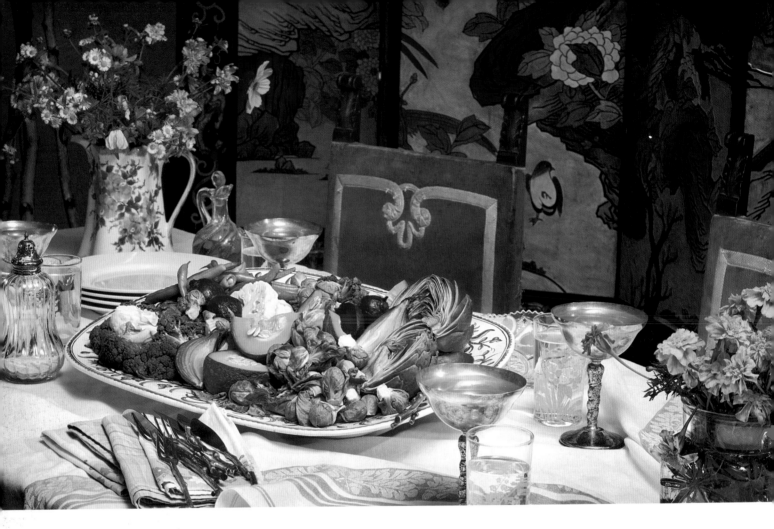

kitchen and from the organic garden and forest at the Wild Woodstock Jivamukti Forest Sanctuary in Woodstock, New York. I hope you enjoy trying out these recipes for yourself and your friends and family. When people cook their own food, they develop more awareness of the connection between what they eat and how they feel.

The great changes in history (such as the abolition of human slavery, women's rights to education and to vote, the end of apartheid in South Africa, and the fall of the Berlin Wall) have never been instigated by governments or corporations but by small groups of committed individuals acting out of consciousness for a greater good. We instigate the awakening of self-confidence within ourselves when we stop blaming others for the ills of the world and instead look at our own lives and ask, "What am I doing to contribute to a more peaceful, joyful, and unpolluted world?" By healing ourselves, we heal the world. After all, the world around us is only a reflection of who we are. And when we make others happy, we become happier too.

To become a vegan is by far the best way we have at this time in history to contribute to peace on Earth. Being a vegan in the world today is to be involved in a nonviolent, direct-action protest against cruelty and an affirmation of kindness. There is no more direct and powerful way to make a positive impact than being vegan. When your grandchildren or great-grandchildren ask you what *you* were doing during the war on Mother Earth, when billions of animals were enslaved, tortured, and exploited as part of the animal holocaust and mass genocide, have you considered what you will tell them? Have the courage to step outside the dictates of an authoritarian world culture that is based on the cruel exploitation of animals and the planet, to joyfully celebrate your respect for yourself and all of life by committing to a diet rooted in kindness. The most courageous act any of us can do at this time is to dare to care about others—other animals, the Earth, and all beings. To be more other-centered rather than self-centered is the first step to happiness. The delicious recipes in this book will not only help you create tasty meals but will help you start your own radical movement of peaceful, joyful coexistence with all of life.

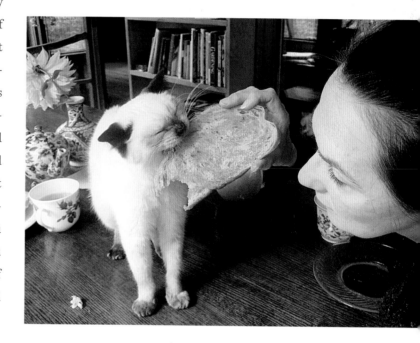

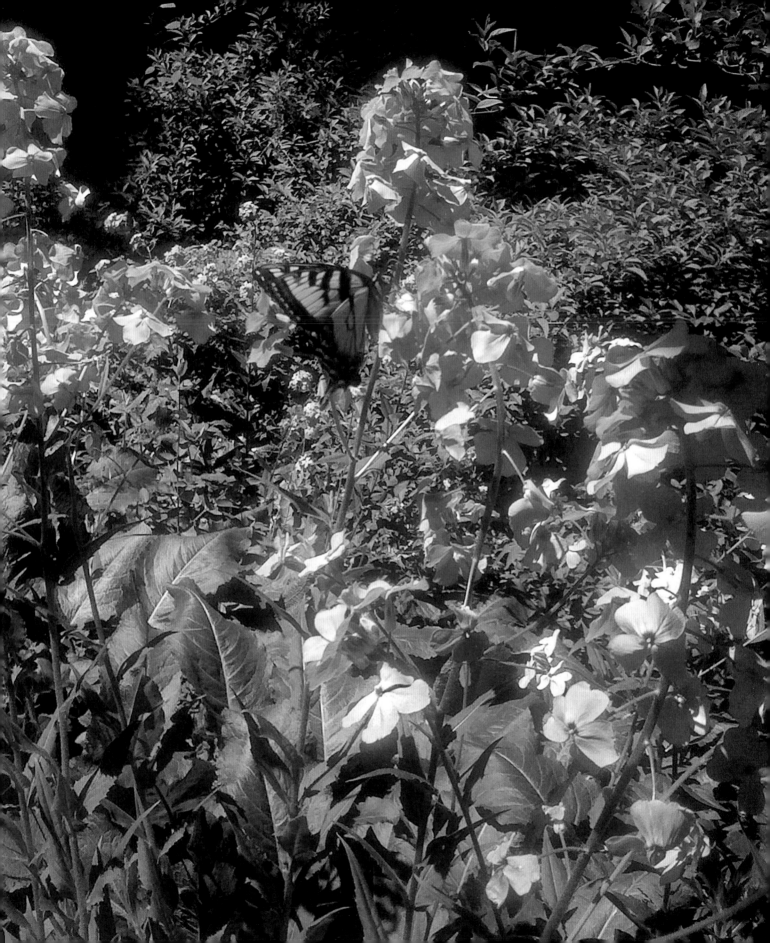

Frequently Asked Questions

WHERE DO I GET MY PROTEIN?

Flesh isn't the only source of protein. You can get all the protein you need from a varied, plant-based diet. Protein is found in greens, vegetables, beans, grains, nuts and seeds, avocados, and so on. And there is no need to consume these foods in any special combination. According to the RDA (recommended daily allowance), we need between 50 and 75 grams of protein per day. Actually, many researchers believe that this number is too high. Look around you. Are Americans suffering from malnourishment? No, we're facing an obesity epidemic. On average, most people consume between 100 and 120 grams of protein per day. Not only is that unhealthy, it's extremely dangerous, as the majority of the protein consumed is animal based. To find out how much protein you need, take your weight (in pounds) and divide it by 3. If you're interested in protein breakdowns and charts, pick up *Becoming Vegan* by Brenda Davis and Vesanto Melina. But rest assured, a varied whole-foods, plant-based diet will give you all the protein you need.

WHAT ABOUT IRON?

According to Dr. Neal Barnard, founder of the Physicians Committee for Responsible Medicine (PCRM), the most healthful sources of iron are leafy greens and beans. These foods also contain calcium and other important minerals. In fact, studies show that vegetarians and vegans tend to get more iron than meat eaters, and vitamin C from fruits and vegetables increases iron absorption.[13] Meanwhile, dairy products reduce iron absorption significantly.[14]

DON'T I NEED TO DRINK MILK TO GET ENOUGH CALCIUM?

No. In fact, drinking milk and eating dairy products can rob your body of calcium and contribute to osteoporosis.[15] The countries that consume the most dairy have the highest rates of hip fracture and osteoporosis.[16] If you eat dark green leafy vegetables like kale, collards, and mustard greens, you can get enough calcium from a vegan diet. Beans, tofu, cabbage, sesame seeds, seaweed, and broccoli are additional sources of calcium. Calcium from vegetable sources is more easily absorbed by the human body than from dairy products.[17]

It's important to understand that calcium isn't just about what you eat; it's also about what you keep. Acidic animal products mine minerals like potassium, magnesium, and calcium from our bodies. If you doubt that you are meeting the 1,000-milligram RDA, include calcium-fortified foods like fruit juice, cereals, or soy or grain beverages, or take a supplement. Also, the weight-bearing aspect of yoga asana practice contributes to bone density and health. Sunlight is essential to the body's ability to absorb calcium from the food you are eating. Make sure you receive adequate vitamin D every day through sunlight. About fifteen to twenty minutes of sun on the face and hands is usually enough for most of us. Read the book *CalciYum!* by David and Rachelle Bronfman for more information.

IS IT OKAY TO DRINK ORGANIC MILK?

Cows that are fed organic food are still kept as slaves on farms, regardless of whether it is a large corporate factory farm or a small family farm. Besides, every dairy cow, no matter what she has been fed, has her babies stolen from her shortly after birth and will inevitably end up in the slaughterhouse.

Milk is for babies. Human beings are the only species that drinks milk into adulthood and prefers to drink the milk of another species (enslaved cows and goats), and we have come to consider it normal when it is actually a pretty perverse form of sexual abuse!

After all, cows can only produce milk when they have been pregnant and given birth, and on dairy farms the only way they can become pregnant is by artificial insemination, which requires a bull to be masturbated and semen to be injected into the cow's vagina, all done by humans.

CAN I GET B$_{12}$ FROM A VEGAN DIET?

A vegan must rely on getting adequate vitamin B$_{12}$ from a supplement or from eating foods that have been fortified with vitamin B$_{12}$. If we weren't so dirt-conscious, we would obtain adequate vitamin B$_{12}$ from soil, air, water, and bacteria, but we meticulously wash and peel our vegetables now—and with good reason, as we can't be sure our soil is not contaminated with pesticides and herbicides. Today "aged" foods like sauerkraut, miso, and tempeh are fermented in hygienically sanitized stainless-steel vats to ensure cleanliness, so we can no longer be sure they will provide us with the B$_{12}$ we need.

Vegans should not mess around with this issue. To ensure that you are getting the tiny amount (2.5 micrograms) you need per day, take a supplement or drink fortified soy milk or rice milk. Read the book *Becoming Vegan* by Brenda Davis and Vesanto Melina for more information.

IF ALL OF LIFE IS SACRED, THEN WHAT IS THE DIFFERENCE IF I EAT A CARROT OR A CHICKEN?

This is a question that often comes up when people have started to consider the morality of imprisoning, abusing, slaughtering, and ultimately eating animals. Yes, all of life is sacred, including plants; and yes, there is research that demonstrates that plants have feelings—they feel it when their leaves or stems are ripped—and there is scientific evidence showing while plants do not have brains and nervous systems like animals, they nevertheless actively work to ensure their survival—they want to live, thrive, reproduce, evolve. If it were possible to live without causing harm to any living being at all, then indeed we might well choose not to eat carrots or other vegetables. But that is not possible—merely by being alive, we necessarily cause harm to many, many beings: we step on them inadvertently, we breathe them in without noticing, we kill them when we brush our teeth or wash our bodies. The best we can do is to strive to minimize the amount of harm we cause by living.

We need to eat in order to live, and there is no moral or ethical code that dictates that we should refrain from eating and allow ourselves to die for some higher purpose. But as humans, we do get to choose what we eat, and when we choose to eat a plant, we are eating (i.e., harming) just that plant, plus indirectly whatever nutrients that plant consumed over its lifetime (and we are also harming whatever beings may have been living on that plant or who were injured or killed in the harvesting process). But when we eat an animal, we are eating not just that animal, but also indirectly all of the plants and other beings that that animal ate over its lifetime—those plants became the flesh that we eat. It takes twelve to twenty pounds of grain (plus one hundred pounds of fish) to produce one pound of beef[18]—that's a lot of harm for one pound of food. And moreover, eating vegetables, fruits, and grains rarely causes total destruction of the plant or tree on which the food grew; after harvesting, seeds remain to be replanted the next season. But this certainly does not happen when an animal is slaughtered—death is final; that animal will not reproduce again!

The imbalance in harm between a plant-based diet and an animal-based diet goes even further. Most of the food crops raised in the world today are fed to livestock destined for slaughter for us to eat, and most of the water used is used to raise the food crops that are fed to those animals. It has been estimated that, because of the extraordinary amount of grain it takes to raise food animals, if we reduced the amount of meat we eat by only 10 percent, enough grain would be freed up to feed all of the starving humans in the world.[19] So when we choose to eat meat instead of plants, we are choosing to take food away from others who are hungry. Additionally, raising crops to feed animals for human consumption requires a lot of land. It takes eight or nine cows annually to feed one average meat eater, and each cow eats one acre of green plants, soybeans, and corn per year, so it takes eight or nine acres of plants a year to feed one meat eater, compared with only half an acre to feed one vegetarian.[20]

Also, most of the plants grown to be fed to farm animals are heavily saturated with pesticides and herbicides and have been genetically modified, all of which contributes to the pollution and destruction of our environment, which harms us all. Intensive farming of the land to grow animal feed, as well as the clearing of forests for grazing animals destined for slaughter, is rapidly ruining the delicate habitats for many wild animals, trees, and wild vegetation.

For all of these reasons, if we want to consider the sanctity of life in deciding what to eat, the choice is clear.

AREN'T HUMANS BIOLOGICALLY DESIGNED TO BE MEAT EATERS OR AT LEAST OMNIVORES?

The anatomical and physiological facts suggest no. We have small, flat mouths with small teeth. We don't have long, sharp canines to tear flesh. We have incisors in the front to bite and molars along the sides to chew and grind fruits and vegetables. Our teeth aren't strong enough to chew and crush hard things like raw bones, whereas carnivores can. We have a rotating jaw that moves from side to side, another useful feature for grinding plants. Carnivores and omnivores have hinge-joint jaws that open and close. They don't normally chew their food well before swallowing, and they don't need to. Unlike us, they don't have an abundance of the enzyme ptyalin in their saliva, which breaks down complex carbohydrates found only in plant foods. Once we have chewed and swallowed our food, it travels through a very long digestive tract, although not as long as that of our herbivore friends—the cows, horses, and sheep. Meat-eating species have comparatively short intestinal tracts, which allow them to move food through their systems quickly, so as not to allow rotting flesh to stagnate and cause disease.

Because we lack sharp claws, aren't very fast on our feet, and aren't exactly endowed with lightning-fast reflexes, it would be very difficult, if not impossible, for us to run down an animal, catch it with our bare hands, and tear through its fur and skin in order to eat it. Biologically, we are designed to be frugivorous herbivores eating mainly fruits, seeds, roots, and leaves.

Humans do not need to eat the flesh of other animals to exist, whereas some animals, like lions and tigers, are carnivores and cannot survive by eating only vegetables. Humans eat meat only out of choice. We have been conditioned, taught, and coerced by the agents of our culture (parents, grandparents, advertisers, food critics, etc.) to eat the flesh and drink the milk of other animals. Because of this conditioning, which has occurred over a long period of time (thousands of years), we have developed addictive eating habits and have blinded ourselves to the facts of our biological system and its true needs.

Many gruesome studies have been done in which cholesterol-rich food was force-fed to dogs and cats in scientific research labs and the results have always proven the same: no matter how much highly saturated animal fat was fed to dogs and cats, it did not affect their arteries—there was no cholesterol built up in their arteries, and the researchers were unable to induce heart disease in them through feeding them a high-protein/high-fat animal flesh diet.[21] This proves that animals like cats and dogs are true omnivores and can eat a wide variety of foods from both animal and vegetable sources. On the other hand, the number of human deaths due to hardening of the arteries and other similar diseases suggests that human beings were not meant to eat animals; our bodies are unable to digest the animal fat effectively and it ends up stored in our blood vessels, not to mention our waistlines, buttocks, and thighs!

Often people will argue about veganism and bring up Eskimos, saying, "Well, what about Eskimos? They have to eat meat to survive—they can't plant vegetable gardens on icebergs." This is true; Arctic-dwelling Eskimos have no choice but to eat large amounts of meat and animal fat. But let's get our facts straight: according to the *American Journal of Clinical Nutrition,* Eskimos also have the highest incidences of heart disease and osteoporosis in the world[22] and, per Geoff Bond in his *Deadly Harvest,* in general they have short life spans.[23] Perhaps that is something to consider when we are faced with the choice of what to eat for dinner; unlike Eskimos, most of us *do* have choices.

In fact, we would know that we are not meant to be meat eaters, and we would not have allowed ourselves to become conditioned to meat eating in the first place, if the effects of meat eating were felt right away. But since heart disease, cancer, diabetes, and osteoporosis usually take many years to develop, we are able to separate them from their cause (or contributing factors) and go on happily eating an animal-based diet. We then become conditioned to see these diseases as occurring normally as we age or as we gain weight or if we eat a "bad diet" (e.g., a diet with *too* much animal products), and we resign ourselves to them and to the expensive and side effect–laden pharmaceutical drug regimens we have devised to deal with them, virtually all of which involve horrendous, sadistic torture to animals in laboratories. We enslave, torture, and then slaughter animals to eat them, then when we eventually become sick from that, we enslave, torture, and kill more animals in laboratories in the hopes of creating drugs to enable us to continue with our animal-abusive lifestyle! Few of us (i.e., our parents and grandparents) look to the future, see the effects of an omnivorous lifestyle, and opt out of it before it makes *us* sick.

ISN'T IT NATURAL TO EAT MEAT? EVEN ANIMALS EAT OTHER ANIMALS. SHOULDN'T WE TRY TO LIVE A MORE NATURAL LIFE?

Some meat eaters defend meat eating by pointing out that it is natural: in the wild, animals eat one another. The animals that end up on our breakfast, lunch, and dinner plates, however, aren't those who normally eat other animals. The animals we exploit for food are not the lions and tigers and bears of the world. For the most part, we eat the gentle, vegan animals. On today's farms, however, we actually force them to become meat eaters by making them eat feed containing the rendered remains of other animals, which they would never eat in the wild.

Lions and other carnivorous animals do eat meat, but that doesn't mean we should. They also live outdoors in all weather, don't wear clothes, don't drive around in cars, and don't shop at grocery stores or farmer's markets. Why cite just one of the many things they do and argue that we should imitate them? This doesn't make much sense. Lions would die if they didn't eat meat. Human beings, in contrast, choose to eat meat; it isn't a physiological necessity. In fact, as mentioned previously, we are designed anatomically to be vegetarians.

HUMAN BEINGS HAVE BEEN EATING MEAT FOREVER. WHY SHOULD WE CHANGE NOW?

There are many activities that human beings have been doing "forever." We might argue from that perspective that eating meat should be allowed to continue. Men have been raping women for thousands of years. Does that mean that it is normal and should be allowed to continue? Human beings have been waging war and destroying the environment for a long time. Just because it has been going on for a long time and become an unquestioned habit, does that mean it should be allowed to continue? Rape, war, slaughtering, and exploiting other animals are not hardwired into us—these are learned behaviors, and that means they can be unlearned. And that's good news! So let's pick up our forks and chopsticks and let the peaceful revolution begin.

Cooking Tips

Here are a few tips to help make your cooking more tasty and nutritious for your body, mind, and spirit, as well as for your greater body—this planet Earth and all the fellow Earthlings that live here with you.

Prayer

Cooking can be a magical act, a potent alchemical process where form transforms into another form. To cultivate the highest intention, pray or chant a mantra before you start to cook, while cooking, and before you eat. To pray is to set a high intention, to implore the Divine forces to come to your aid for a good and selfless end. As you approach the cooking process and then the eating of the food you have cooked, make sure that your mind and heart are centered in a high intentional mood. This will purify the whole experience, ridding the kitchen of subtle toxins like anger and impatience.

See the entire process—from thinking about what to cook, to gathering and preparing the ingredients, to the actual cooking, to eating your food, and ultimately to cleaning up before and afterward—as a devotional offering that will not only please yourself and others but God as well. See your kitchen area as part of God's abode, as sacred space, as a doorway to enlightenment. Your kitchen is a temple and all the pots, pans, spices, grains, fruits, and vegetables, as well as the stove, spoons, knives, bowls, and plates, are all Divine objects, full of consciousness, waiting to become part of the Divine alchemical process of creating a meal. Treat them with respect, like you would your guru or esteemed teacher; view them as your partners, for they will help carry your soulful intentions to the Supreme Self. Allow the fire of your soul to become part of the heating element that cooks your food.

Many of us in the West are familiar with the practice of saying grace before eating, yet many modern people feel this is old-fashioned, superstitious, or devoid of any true significance. Most feel it is unnecessary to even thank Mother Earth for food but rather feel entitled to it. Yet in the yogic tradition, offering food to God first, before eating, is a fundamental practice that is incorporated into daily life.

In the Bhagavad Gita, an ancient Indian text, Krishna gives advice to the wannabe yogi, Arjuna, saying that if you want to dispel ignorance and anxiety, do what you do but remember God when you are doing it— offer all of your actions to God, even the food you eat. *"Pattram pushpam phalam toyam / yo me bhaktya prayacchati / tad aham bhakti-upahritam / ashnami prayata-atmanah."* "Whatever is offered to me with a pure loving heart, no matter if it is a leaf, a flower, fruit, or a sip of water, I will accept it. The one who remembers me is dear to me" (Bhagavad Gita 9.26).

Food, drink, or even water that has first been offered to God is known in the Sanskrit

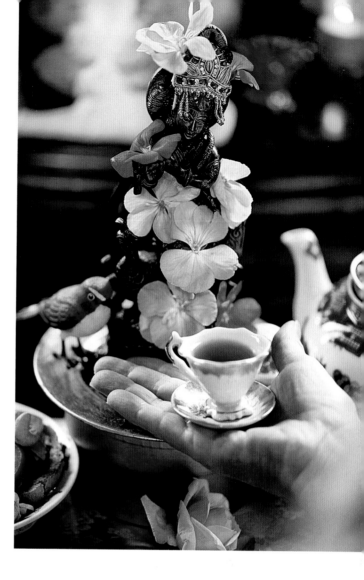

language as *prasad*, which literally means "a gracious blessed gift." In fact, the yogic tradition suggests that you should never consume anything that has not first been offered to God, because if you ingest unoffered food, you are possibly ingesting selfishness and unconsciousness, and that will have an effect on your own physical, mental, emotional, and ultimately spiritual well-being. Eating offered food, on the other hand, assures that you will have a Divine dining experience because *prasad* contains the deity's blessing within it. Eating *prasad* allows you to cultivate more consciousness of what you are eating. You are less likely to be driven by appetite cravings and mechanically just stuff your mouth. Instead, you take time and prepare the food as a gift, not for yourself but for God. The time among preparing, offering, and then eating the food allows devotion, the remembrance of God, to be cultivated. Traditionally, the cooking and preparing of food is done without tasting by the cook because the food should be offered to God first and then consumed. In this way, eating *prasad* is thought of as eating God's leftovers. One way that food can be offered is to place the prepared food on a plate, in a bowl, or in a cup in front of an image or statue of a spiritual deity and ask for the intention of our devotion to be accepted by God and for the food to be transformed into blessed *prasad*, ready to be eaten. Another way is to mentally offer the food by saying a prayer over the plate before eating.

My friend Shyamdas, who was an enlightened master in the ways of cultivating joy and spiritual devotion (*bhakti*) through the practice of cooking and who was my teacher in such things, told me that "all the food that you prepare should be first offered to God, then shared with other *bhaktas*, then finally eaten yourself. In this way, your own spiritual devotion is sure to increase."

True, it may not be practical to have dinner guests every night, but you can at least spend a moment to say a prayer of offering over your food before you eat it and find someone to give a spoonful of your meal to—maybe your dog or cat or a bird who may visit your windowsill. Or if there really is no one else around to share the food with, you can always make a mental offering to someone else, even a loved one who has passed on. The point is, in order to cultivate sacredness around eating, you should try at least to be thankful for your food and share your food with others—not just eat to satisfy your own appetite. It is said in the yogic tradition that eating offered food regularly changes the actual cells and tissues of your body, resulting in a refined, lighter, more spiritual body—with skin that literally exudes a glow.

If you are in a bad mood, it is best to stay out of the kitchen. If there are other people in the kitchen with you while you are preparing food, don't engage in mundane talk, idle chitchat, or gossip with them, as this will affect the food vibrationally. It is best to keep off-point conversation out of the kitchen while preparing food and keep talking to a minimum or remain silent and chant mantras silently to yourself while preparing food. If you have a CD or iPod player in the kitchen, it can be helpful to play recorded music of mantras or uplifting spiritual music while preparing food.

Most of us in the West understand offering food to God as saying grace over a meal, and that can manifest from a very simple expression of gratitude over your food before you eat it to very elaborate rituals. Here are two Sanskrit mantras from the yogic tradition that can be used as blessings to offer your food with the highest spiritual intention, which will in turn infuse your food with spiritual potency and manifest in your well-being:

Lokah Samastah Sukhino Bhavantu
Om Shantih Shantih Shantih Hari Om

Translation: May all beings be happy and free, and may the thoughts, words, and actions of my own life contribute in some way to that happiness and to that freedom for all. Peace, Peace, Peace to all existence.

Brahmarpanam Brahma-Havir
Brahmagnau Brahmana Hutam
Brahmaiva Tena Gantavyam
Brahma-Karma-Samadhina
BHAGAVAD GITA 4.24

Translation: See God (Brahman) everywhere: God is the ladle; God also is the food; God is the fire; God is the preparer; and God is the eater of the food. God is the reason for eating and God is the goal to be reached.

When mantras like these are used as a blessing over food, the result is that the preparing of the meal, the ones who are preparing and offering the meal, and the eating of the offered meal all become merged and the experience exudes a magical potency that can actually bring one closer to the knowledge of the transcendental Divine Reality. The so-called simple act of preparing and eating food *can be* a spiritual experience if the intention is there.

Garlic and Onions

Many yogis, Vaishnavas (worshippers of Lord Vishnu and his incarnations), and high-caste Indian Brahmins abstain from eating garlic and onions. While there are many reasons for this restriction, essentially the thought is that eating garlic and onions affects your consciousness in such a way as to inhibit meditation. Garlic and onions are considered rajasic and are thought to induce passion, not tranquillity, in the mind. In the Indian ayurvedic system, garlic and onions are used medicinally and not in daily fare because, if eaten regularly, their medicinal potency is diminished. In the ancient Vedic culture, garlic and onions were used in the cooking of meat, so to the Indian mind they are associated with meat eating. In the caste system of India, the highest caste are Brahmins and they are traditionally vegetarians who do not eat garlic and onions, whereas the other, lower castes are not so restrictive with their food and often include meat and garlic and onions, whether they are preparing vegetarian or meat-based dishes. So the use of garlic and onions could also be viewed from a class or caste perspective.

Personally, I don't eat much garlic and onions, but I am not strictly against their use. I am more concerned with veganism and don't mind if people need to "spice up" their vegetables with garlic and onions. There are many recipes in this book that use garlic and onions, but if you prefer, consider them optional and leave them out of the recipe.

Hygiene

Before preparing food, wash your hands thoroughly and also remove any jewelry you may be wearing on your fingers, hands, and wrists because bacteria and dirt can hide in the jewelry and be transferred into the food. Remove all fingernail polish for this same reason. Tie back your hair or contain it in a hairnet or hat so that hair does not fall into the food you are preparing. The kitchen should be clean, including all countertops and cutting boards, as well as the floor, before preparation of the food is begun.

Pots and Pans

Never use aluminum cooking pots or aluminum foil or Teflon pans. Instead, use cast iron, stainless steel, glass, or enamel (if it isn't chipped). Teflon-coated aluminum pots and pans can become toxic because, over time with use, the Teflon will chip off and get into the food; this is especially true if you use metal spoons, forks, or spatulas when cooking, which scratch the surface of the pan.

To Boil or Steam?

When vegetables are boiled, a lot of the nutrients leach into the cooking water. If that water is discarded, then those nutrients are lost. Steaming is the best way to keep nutrients from being lost in the cooking process.

It is a good idea to invest in a couple of different steamers. I use stainless steel. I have one that looks like a large soup pot with two baskets that fit inside, one very deep and one shallow, which fits on top of the deeper one. I can steam potatoes and yams in the deep bottom one while I steam greens in the top. I also have a small collapsible one that fits inside almost any size of pot. I use it when I just want to steam a small amount and don't want to pull out the big one.

Remember: when you are steaming, you don't need to fill the steaming pan with a lot of water. The waterline should be below the vegetables. Make sure there is enough water in the pan so that it won't all evaporate before you are finished steaming your vegetables; otherwise, you will be left with a dry pot burning on the stove.

Oils

Always use organic and cold-pressed oils. It is always best not to cook oils; instead, consume them raw. When certain oils are heated, their molecular structure is altered and, as a result, toxic products are formed that can damage the liver and kidneys and lead to premature aging of the body and even cancer. The oils that resist heat destruction the best are olive oil, coconut oil, sunflower oil, safflower oil, and canola oil.

Deep-fried foods should be avoided, because (1) the oil is heated to a very high temperature, making it difficult and harmful for your body to digest, and (2) it takes a large amount of oil to deep-fry food and, because of that, the oil is usually used over and over again and reheated each time. This alters the oil chemically and produces free radicals, which can be a health hazard.[24]

Sautéing food in oil is better than deep-frying. If you are planning to sauté, use olive oil, coconut oil, sunflower oil, safflower oil, or canola oil. But make sure that the oil you use is organic and not genetically modified (GMO). About half of the nonorganic canola oil is made from genetically modified crops, and most of the corn oil as well, so be sure to buy organic. Flaxseed oil, which is the most unsaturated, should always be consumed raw and never be subjected to heat. *You should never cook with flaxseed oil.*

Vegans should aim for 15 to 30 percent of the calories consumed daily to be from fat in the form of unprocessed oils, nuts, seeds, raw nut butters, olives, soy milk, coconut, and avocados. Avoid hydrogenated fats in the form of margarine, deep-fried foods (French fries), and chips. There are some vegan margarines available that are not made with hydrogenated fats—read the labels.

Salt and Pepper

In most of my recipes I prefer to add salt and pepper at the end before serving, because salt tends to inhibit the molecular breakdown of the food. This is especially true when cooking beans and lentils, which can remain hard.

A Well-Stocked Kitchen Should Have . . .

Pots, Pans, Appliances, and Utensils

Double-decker stainless-steel steamer

Double-decker double boiler

Large soup pot with thick bottom

2 medium saucepans with tight-fitting lids

2 small saucepans with tight-fitting lids

1 large Dutch oven (thick-walled cooking pot or casserole dish with a tight-fitting lid)

1 large cast-iron frying pan

1 medium frying pan

1 small frying pan

Glass baking dishes in assorted sizes

Pie and cake pans

Several cutting boards—bamboo or plastic (but if you are going to buy the plastic kind, don't buy white; get the colored ones because they won't stain and look dirty after a few uses!)

Knives, assorted—best to have knives where the metal goes all the way into the end of the handle

Scissors, used only for cutting vegetables

Vegetable peeler

Measuring cups for dry ingredients

Tempered-glass measuring cups for liquids

Measuring spoons

Tongs

Soup ladle

Pasta claw (stainless steel or wood is best)

2 wire-mesh strainers, one small and one large

Heavy-duty blender (Vitamix brand is best)

Handheld immersion blender

Large food processor (able to accommodate at least 9 cups)

Mortar and pestle (for grinding herbs and spices)

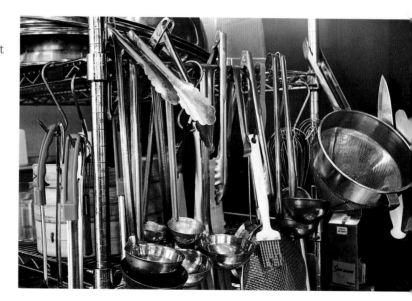

Food Staples—Dry (Unrefrigerated), Organic to the Extent Possible

Brown rice

Millet

Quinoa

Kasha (buckwheat groats)

Oatmeal

Red lentils

Green lentils

Dried split peas

Assorted noodles and pasta

Pastry flour

All-purpose flour

Raw, unprocessed sugar

Agave

Powdered egg replacer (such as Ener-G brand)

Cocoa powder, unsweetened

Raw cacao

Nutritional yeast flakes

Powdered spirulina

Vanilla extract

Almond extract

Vegan powdered soup broth and/or bouillon cubes

Ground cumin

Ground coriander

Ground cinnamon

Ground ginger

Powdered garlic

Powdered onion

Cayenne pepper

Black sesame seeds

Salt

Freshly ground black pepper

Olive oil

Coconut oil

Toasted sesame oil

Balsamic vinegar

White vinegar

Apple cider vinegar

Canned tomato sauce

Canned coconut milk

Soy sauce (shoyu), tamari (wheat-free soy sauce) and/or Braggs Liquid Aminos (unfermented soy sauce)

Dried seaweed, assorted (hijiki, kombu, arame, wakame, and agar-agar flakes)

Dried and canned beans, assorted (black, garbanzos, adzuki, black-eyed peas, cannellini, pinto, and kidney)

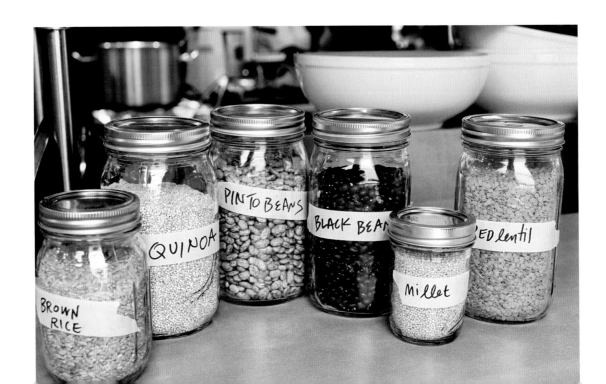

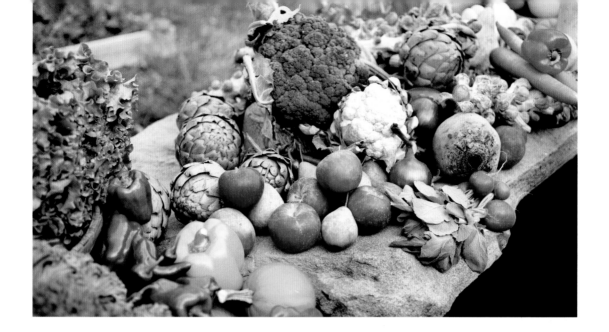

Food Staples—Fresh or Refrigerated Foods, Organic to the Extent Possible

Margarine (such as Earth Balance brand, available in the United States)

Flaxseed oil

Soy milk

Almond milk

Dijon mustard

Veganaise (commercially prepared vegan mayonnaise)

Lemons

Garlic

Onions

Potatoes

Yams

Parsley

Lettuce / assorted salad greens

Kale

Cabbage

Apples

Carrots

Celery

Measurement Conversions

$\frac{1}{8}$ teaspoon = a pinch

1 tablespoon = 3 teaspoons

2 tablespoons = $\frac{1}{8}$ cup

4 tablespoons = $\frac{1}{4}$ cup

8 tablespoons = $\frac{1}{2}$ cup

12 tablespoons = $\frac{3}{4}$ cup

16 tablespoons = 1 cup

1 cup = 8 fluid ounces

2 cups = 1 pint = 16 fluid ounces

4 cups = 2 pints = 1 quart

16 cups = 8 pints = 4 quarts = 1 gallon

U.S. to Metric Conversions (Approximate)

$\frac{1}{5}$ teaspoon = 1 milliliter

1 teaspoon = 5 milliliters

1 tablespoon = 15 milliliters

1 fluid ounce = 30 milliliters

$\frac{1}{5}$ cup = 50 milliliters

1 cup = 240 milliliters

2 cups = 1 pint = 470 milliliters

4 cups = 1 quart = 0.95 liter

4.2 cups = 2.1 pints = 1 liter

1.06 quarts = 0.26 gallon = 1 liter

4 quarts = 1 gallon = 3.8 liters

1 ounce = 28 grams

1 pound = 454 grams

2.205 pounds = 35 ounces = 1 kilogram

Oven Temperature Conversions— Fahrenheit to Celsius (Approximate)

275°F = 135°C

300°F = 150°C

325°F = 165°C

350°F = 180°C

375°F = 190°C

400°F = 200°C

425°F = 220°C

450°F = 230°C

475°F = 250°C

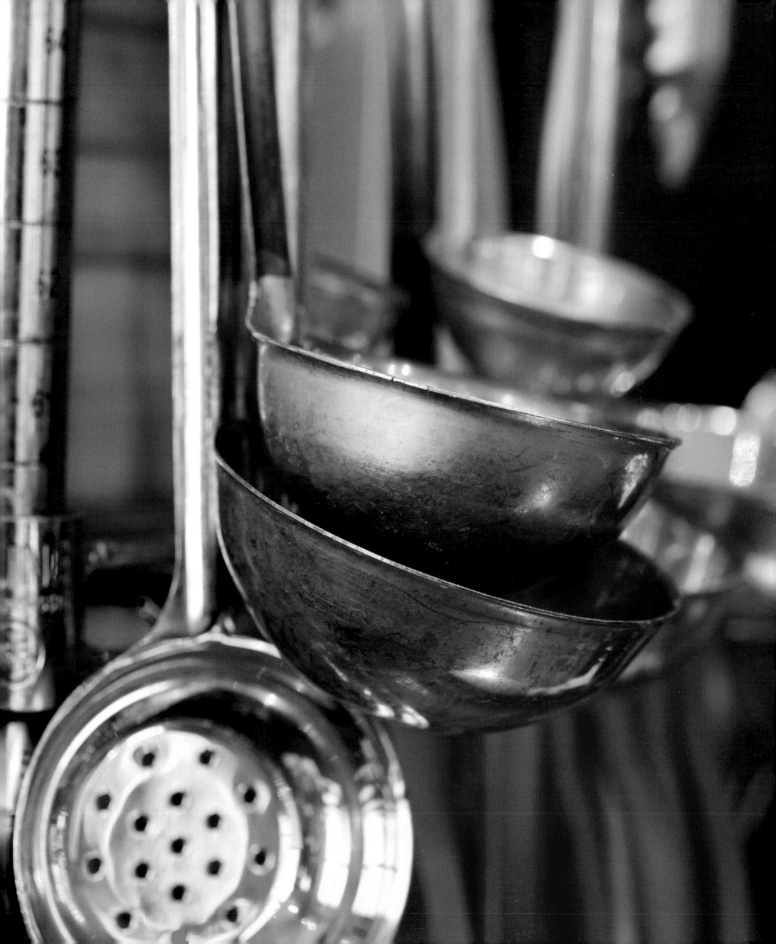

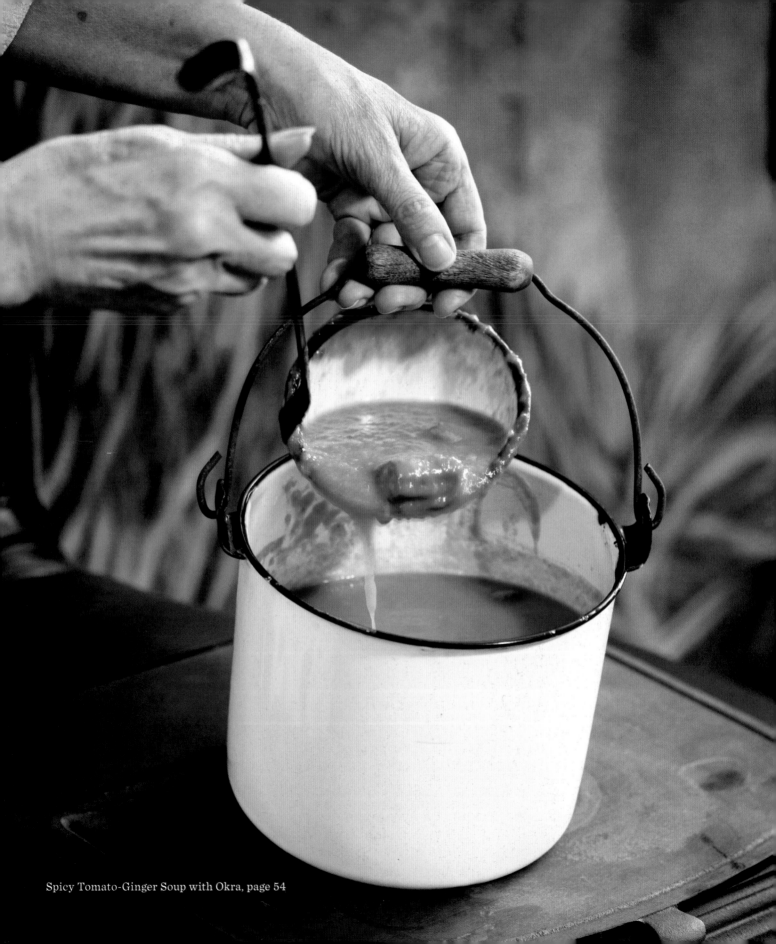

Spicy Tomato-Ginger Soup with Okra, page 54

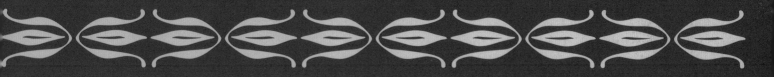

Soups

Vegetable soups consist of one or more kinds of vegetables combined with water and/or vegetable stock or nondairy milk. Soups can be served hot or cold, and the ingredients can be cooked or raw. Soups are versatile and can be served as a main entrée or as a starter or side dish. For some people, eating a variety of vegetables served separately is challenging to the digestion, but when they are combined into a soup, their digestibility is enhanced. By far the greatest number of recipes in this cookbook are soup recipes, organized into six basic types according to texture: blended, creamy, chunky, noodle, broth, and raw. Most of these recipes produce a hearty consistency; feel free to add water or other liquid if you prefer a lighter soup.

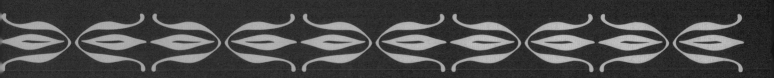

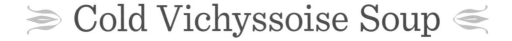

Cold Vichyssoise Soup

Here is the classic French chilled summer soup, made vegan.

¼ cup olive oil

1 onion, chopped

½ pound crimini mushrooms

2 tablespoons dried tarragon

6 medium potatoes, unpeeled and
chopped into small pieces

½ head celery (6 to 8 stalks with leaves),
chopped into small pieces

3 tablespoons powdered vegetable
stock or equivalent in bouillon cubes,
dissolved in ½ cup boiling water

8 to 10 cups water, depending on
desired consistency

½ cup dry white wine (optional)

Salt and freshly ground black pepper to
taste

Potato chips, for serving

In a medium frying pan, heat the olive oil over medium heat. Add the onion, mushrooms, and tarragon and sauté for 5 to 10 minutes, until the onions are translucent.

In a large soup pot, place the potatoes, celery, sautéed mixture, stock, and water and bring to a boil over high heat. Boil rapidly for 5 minutes. Reduce the heat to medium-low and cook for 45 minutes. Add the wine, if using, and salt and pepper to taste. Cool the soup in the refrigerator for at least 6 hours or overnight. When ready to serve, pour the soup into a blender jar (or use an immersion blender) and blend to a creamy consistency. Ladle the soup into individual bowls, and garnish with a few potato chips floating on top.

SERVES 8 TO 10

Creamy Coconut-Zucchini Soup

The fired-up combination of earthy, watery zucchini and airy,
tropical coconut makes for an elemental sensation.

3 to 6 zucchini, depending on their size,
cut into ½-inch slices

6 medium potatoes, unpeeled and
chopped into small pieces

8 cups water

6 lemons, peeled, seeds and core
removed

One 10- to 15-ounce can coconut milk

½ cup coconut oil

½ cup dry white wine (optional)

3 tablespoons fresh tarragon

1 tablespoon salt

½ teaspoon freshly ground black
pepper

Potato chips, for serving

In a steamer basket, place the zucchini and steam for about 20 minutes, until soft. Set aside.

In a large soup pot, place the potatoes and the water and bring to a boil over high heat. Reduce the heat to medium and cook the potatoes until soft, about 15 minutes.

Using a slotted spoon, remove the potatoes from the pot (reserve the water) and put them into the bowl of a food processor along with the zucchini and lemons. Blend well, adding some of the potato cooking liquid as needed for a smooth consistency. (If using an immersion blender, add the zucchini and lemons, and blend in the pot.) Add the coconut milk, coconut oil, wine, if using, tarragon, salt, and pepper and blend until creamy. When ready to serve, ladle the soup into individual bowls and garnish with a few potato chips floating on top. This soup can also be served cold.

SERVES 8 TO 10

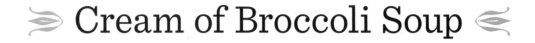 Cream of Broccoli Soup

The use of split peas instead of cream provides not only the creamy texture but also a nutty flavor, a deeper green color, and a boost in the protein content.

3 cups dried split peas

12 cups water

1 onion, chopped

6 cloves garlic, chopped

3 stalks celery, chopped

3 large heads broccoli, including stems
 and florets, chopped

Salt to taste

Soak the peas in cold water for at least 4 hours or overnight. Drain and rinse the peas, then place them in a large soup pot. Add the water and bring to a boil over high heat. Reduce the heat to medium-low and continue to cook, partially covered, for $2\frac{1}{2}$ hours. Add the onion, garlic, celery, and broccoli to the pot and cook until the vegetables are soft and the soup develops a creamy, gravy-like consistency, about 30 minutes.

Place the soup into the bowl of a food processor (or use an immersion blender) and blend. Add salt to taste.

SERVES 12 TO 14

≋ Cream of Celery Soup ≋

In Woodstock, we usually grow a big bed of celery and the forest provides us with an abundance of wild mushrooms, so I usually make this soup in the fall around harvesttime.

1 large head celery, stalks and leaves, chopped

4 medium Yellow Finn potatoes (or any variety), unpeeled and chopped into small pieces

1 bunch fresh parsley, finely chopped

1 carrot, peeled and chopped into small pieces

10 cups water

1 ounce dried mushrooms, any kind

2 tablespoons olive oil

4 cloves garlic, finely chopped

1 tablespoon dried tarragon

1 tablespoon dried thyme

One 10- to 15-ounce can coconut milk, or 2 cups soy milk or almond milk

Salt and freshly ground black pepper to taste

In a large soup pot, place the celery, potatoes, parsley, carrot, and water and bring the mixture to a rapid boil over high heat. Reduce the heat to medium-low and cook for about 45 minutes, or until the vegetables are soft.

Meanwhile, in a small bowl, place the mushrooms, add boiling water to cover, and let stand for 5 to 10 minutes to rehydrate. Drain the mushrooms and set aside, reserving the soaking liquid.

In a medium frying pan, heat the olive oil over medium heat. Add the garlic, tarragon, and thyme and sauté for 3 minutes. Add the rehydrated mushrooms and cook for 5 more minutes, then add the vegetable mixture and the mushroom soaking liquid to the soup pot, stirring well. Let the soup cool slightly, then transfer the soup to the bowl of a food processor and blend well (or use an immersion blender). Return the soup to the pot. Stir in the coconut milk and salt and pepper to taste and simmer for 5 more minutes.

SERVES 10 TO 12

⋙ Creamy Wild ⋘
Mushroom Soup

The sweet, light, and tart applesauce contrasts with the rich
and savory mushrooms to provide an unexpected lift.

1 cup dried wild hen-of-the-woods
    (maitake) mushrooms
6 potatoes (Yellow Finn or red work
    best), unpeeled and cut into small
    pieces
8 cups water
2 tablespoons olive oil
4 cloves garlic, chopped
1 tablespoon dried rosemary

1 tablespoon dried thyme
1 tablespoon powdered vegetable stock
    or equivalent in bouillon cubes,
    dissolved in ¼ cup boiling water
1 tablespoon salt
½ teaspoon freshly ground black
    pepper
One 12-ounce jar organic applesauce

In a small bowl, place the mushrooms and add boiling water to cover. Let stand for 5 to 10 minutes to rehydrate then drain the mushrooms, reserving the soaking liquid.

Place the potatoes in a large soup pot. Add the water and bring to a boil over high heat. Reduce the heat to medium and cook until the potatoes become soft, about 15 minutes.

In a large frying pan, heat the olive oil over medium heat. Add the rehydrated mushrooms, garlic, rosemary, and thyme and sauté for about 5 minutes, until the mushrooms are soft. Pour the mushroom soaking liquid into a measuring cup and add enough potato cooking water to make 1 cup. Add the liquid, stock, salt, and pepper to the frying pan, reduce the heat to low, cover the pan, and simmer for 10 minutes.

In the bowl of a food processor (or using an immersion blender), blend the potatoes and half the sautéed ingredients until smooth and creamy, adding some potato cooking water if necessary to achieve the desired consistency. Stir in the remaining sautéed ingredients. Ladle the soup into individual bowls and garnish each with a large spoonful of cold applesauce.

SERVES 8 TO 10

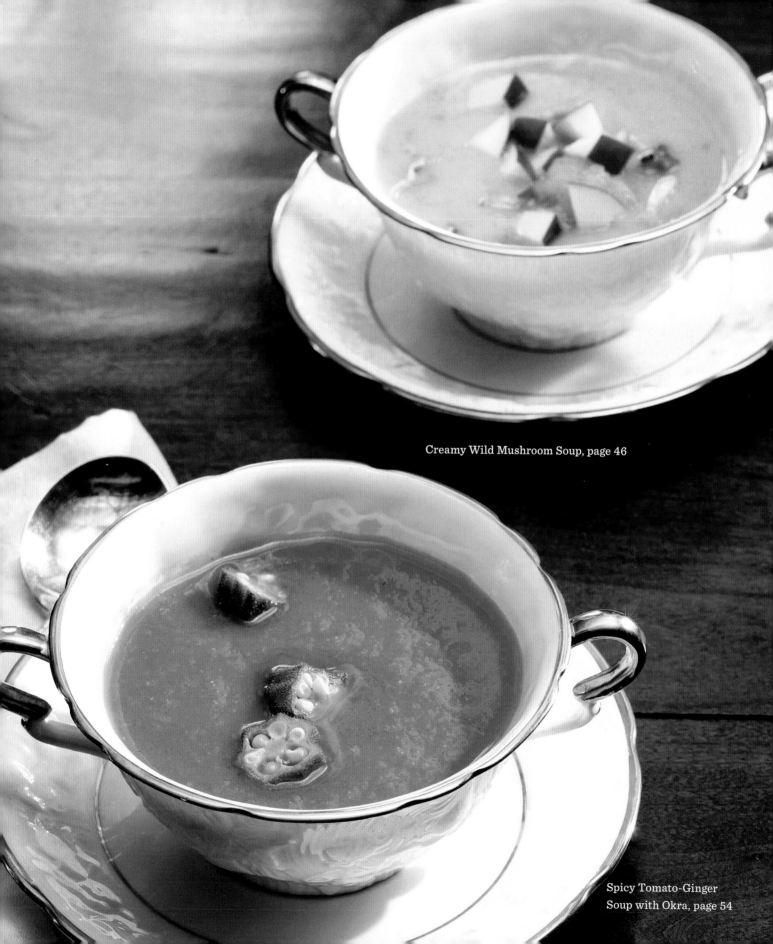

Creamy Wild Mushroom Soup, page 46

Spicy Tomato-Ginger
Soup with Okra, page 54

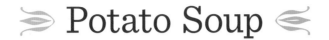 Potato Soup

Potatoes are one of the easiest vegetables for an amateur gardener to grow and usually provide a good yield, which means we eat lots of soup in the fall. The potato chips introduce a texture that the blending takes away.

¼ cup olive oil

1 onion, chopped

½ pound crimini or portabella mushrooms, chopped

2 tablespoons dried tarragon

1 tablespoon dried thyme

8 medium potatoes (any variety), unpeeled and chopped

8 stalks celery with leaves, chopped

8 to 10 cups water, depending on desired consistency

3 tablespoons powdered vegetable stock or equivalent in bouillon cubes, dissolved in ½ cup boiling water

1 cup coconut milk, soy milk, or almond milk

Salt and freshly ground black pepper to taste

Potato chips (vinegar or salt-and-pepper flavor is preferable), for serving

In a medium frying pan, heat the olive oil over medium-high heat. Add the onion, mushrooms, tarragon, and thyme and sauté for 5 to 10 minutes, until the onions are translucent.

Meanwhile, in a large soup pot, place the potatoes and celery, add the water, and bring to a boil over high heat. Boil rapidly for 5 minutes. Reduce the heat to medium-low. Add the stock and the sautéed onion mixture to the pot and cook, covered, for 45 minutes. Add the coconut milk and salt and pepper to taste.

Transfer the soup to the bowl of a food processor and blend well (or use an immersion blender). Ladle the soup into individual bowls and garnish with potato chips.

SERVES 8 TO 10

Potato-Leek Soup

You won't notice the absence of cream in this simple-to-make, traditional comfort food.

6 medium potatoes, peeled and chopped

2 tablespoons powdered vegetable stock or equivalent in bouillon cubes, dissolved in ½ cup boiling water

2 leeks (white and light green parts only), chopped

8 cups water

2 tablespoons olive oil

2 cloves garlic, finely chopped

1 bunch fresh parsley, finely chopped

1 tablespoon dried tarragon

Salt and freshly ground black pepper to taste

In a large soup pot, place the potatoes, stock, leeks, and water and bring to a boil over high heat. Reduce the heat to medium-low and cook for 35 minutes.

Meanwhile, in a small frying pan, heat the olive oil over medium heat. Add the garlic, parsley, and tarragon and sauté for 3 minutes. Add the sautéed garlic mixture to the pot and cook, covered, for 15 more minutes. Place the soup in the bowl of a food processor and blend until smooth (or use an immersion blender). Add salt and pepper to taste.

SERVES 6 TO 10

⋑ Quick-and-Easy ⋐ Cream of Tomato Soup

In five minutes or less, you can be enjoying a warm bowl of comfort.

One 8-ounce can tomato sauce
Water, as needed to reach the
    desired consistency

¼ cup soy milk, almond milk,
    rice milk, or coconut milk
Salt and freshly ground black
    pepper to taste

In a medium saucepan, combine the tomato sauce and enough water to yield the desired consistency. Bring to a boil over high heat and boil for 2 minutes. Add the soy milk and salt and pepper to taste.

SERVES 2 TO 4

Deluxe Cream of Tomato Soup

This is a more robust version of the Quick-and-Easy Cream of Tomato Soup (page 50). It requires a little more preparation, but the results speak for themselves.

1 tablespoon ground cumin

1 tablespoon powdered vegetable stock or equivalent in bouillon cubes, dissolved in ¼ cup boiling water

2 tablespoons vegetable oil

1 large onion, chopped

2 tablespoons pastry flour (or use brown rice flour for a gluten-free soup)

One 22-ounce can or jar tomato sauce

1 teaspoon salt, plus more to taste

½ teaspoon freshly ground black pepper, plus more to taste

1 tablespoon brown rice syrup or sugar

1 cup soy milk, almond milk, or coconut milk

1 to 2 cups water, depending on desired consistency

Dissolve the cumin in the stock and set aside.

In a medium frying pan, heat the vegetable oil over medium-high heat. Add the onion and sauté for 5 to 10 minutes, until translucent. Using a fork, alternately stir in small amounts of flour and stock to make a thin gravy, adding more water if necessary. In the bowl of a food processor, place the gravy, tomato sauce, salt, pepper, brown rice syrup, and soy milk and blend well.

In a medium soup pot, combine the blended mixture with the water. (If using an immersion blender, place all of the ingredients in a medium soup pot and blend well.) Bring the soup to a boil over high heat, stirring often. Remove from the heat. Add salt and pepper to taste.

SERVES 4 TO 6

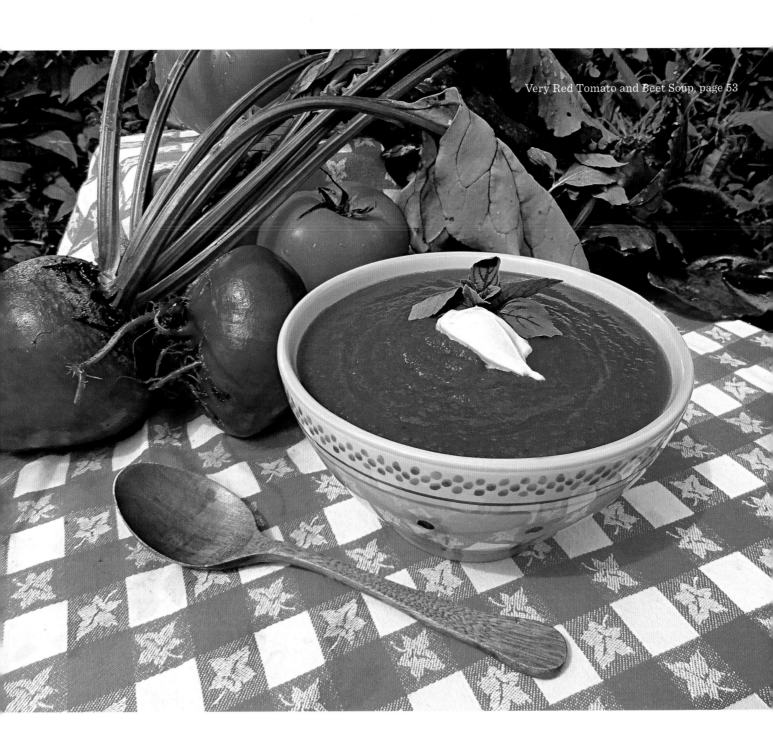

Very Red Tomato and Beet Soup, page 53

⇒ Very Red Tomato ⇐ and Beet Soup

Adding a root vegetable like beets to a tomato soup mellows the tomatoes and deepens the color. Red is the color of the root chakra, so this soup is grounding. Red is also known to increase the appetite, so consider doubling the recipe!

2 large fresh beets, peeled and chopped

One 22-ounce can or jar tomato sauce

2 to 3 cups water, depending on desired consistency

Salt and freshly ground black pepper to taste

Tofu sour cream (optional), for serving

In a large soup pot, place the beets and tomato sauce, add the water and bring to a boil over high heat. Reduce the heat to medium-low and cook for about 30 minutes, until the beets are soft.

Place the soup in the bowl of a food processor and blend until smooth (or use an immersion blender). Transfer the soup back into the pot, add salt and pepper to taste, and reheat if necessary. Ladle the soup into individual bowls and garnish with tofu sour cream, if desired.

SERVES 4 TO 6

Spicy Tomato-Ginger Soup

The ginger provides an unexpected kick to this already spicy soup.

2 tablespoons vegetable oil

1 large potato, unpeeled and chopped
  into small pieces

1 large onion, chopped

1 stalk celery, chopped

One ½-inch piece fresh ginger, peeled
  and chopped

1½ teaspoons ground cumin

1 teaspoon salt

⅛ teaspoon cayenne pepper

1 tablespoon powdered vegetable stock
  or equivalent in bouillon cubes,
  dissolved in ¼ cup boiling water

One 22-ounce can or jar tomato sauce

2 to 3 cups water, depending on desired
  consistency

Vegan sour cream, for serving

3 sprigs fresh cilantro or parsley, finely
  chopped, for serving

In a large frying pan, heat the vegetable oil over medium-high heat. Add the potato, onion, celery, and ginger to the pan. Sprinkle with the cumin, salt, and cayenne and sauté until the onions are golden. Add the stock, reduce the heat to medium-low, and simmer for 10 minutes.

Transfer the mixture to a large soup pot, add the tomato sauce and water, and cook for 20 minutes over medium heat.

Place the soup in the bowl of a food processor and blend until smooth (or use an immersion blender). Ladle the soup into individual bowls and garnish with a spoonful of vegan sour cream and chopped cilantro.

VARIATION

This soup can be made into Tomato-Okra Soup by adding 1 pound fresh or frozen precooked okra, sliced into ¼-inch pieces, after blending.

SERVES 4 TO 6

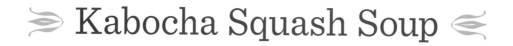 Kabocha Squash Soup

Chinese five-spice powder provides this classic Asian soup a distinctive elegance.

1 medium kabocha squash, chopped

1 cup cooked brown or white rice

¼ cup miso paste (red or golden),
    dissolved in 1 cup boiling water

1 tablespoon Chinese five-spice powder

One 10- to 15-ounce can coconut milk

6 to 8 cups water, depending on desired
    consistency

Steam the squash for about 20 minutes, until soft. When the squash has cooled enough, remove the skin.

Place the squash, rice, miso, five-spice powder, and coconut milk in the bowl of a food processor and blend well, adding a little water as needed to reach a smooth consistency (or use an immersion blender). In a large soup pot, bring the water to a boil and stir in the blended squash mixture.

SERVES 8 TO 10

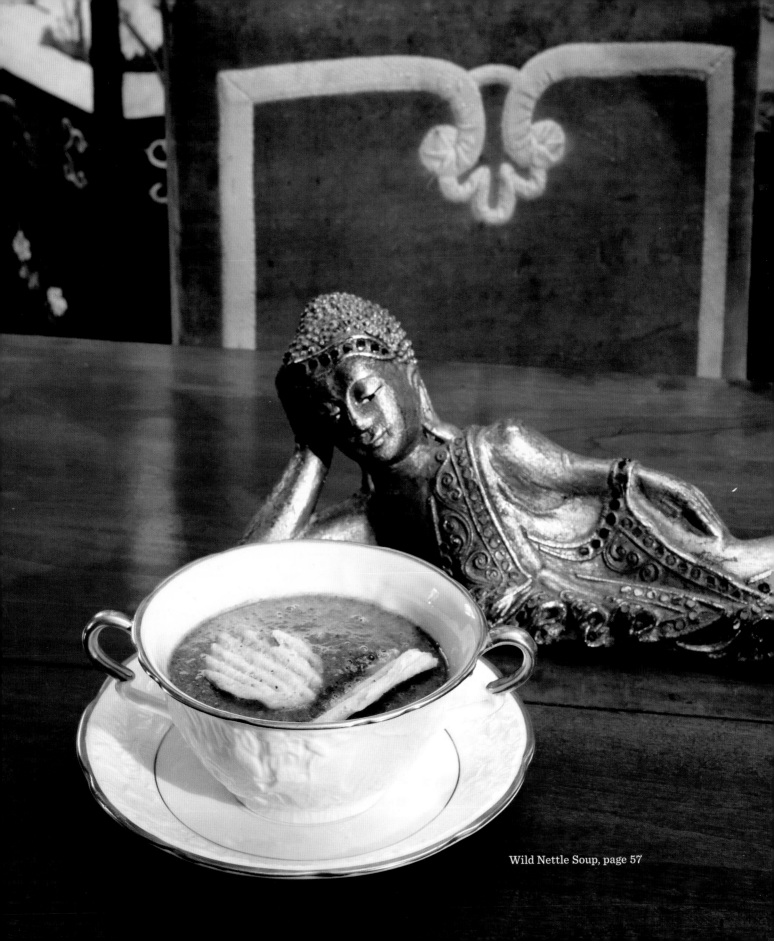

Wild Nettle Soup, page 57

⇒ Wild Nettle Soup ⇐

As legend has it, Tibet's well-known eleventh-century yogi Milarepa lived
exclusively on a diet of nettles. Nettles provide one of the greatest concentrations
of protein in the vegetable world, which is saying a lot for a green leaf. I am very fortunate
to have wild nettles growing in my backyard in Woodstock. I make gallons of this
soup in the spring and freeze it so we can enjoy it throughout the year.

2 tablespoons olive oil

1 large onion, chopped

1 tablespoon dried tarragon

½ pound stinging nettle leaves (use
rubber gloves to remove the leaves
from the stems because they do
sting)

1 large potato, unpeeled and chopped

3 tablespoons powdered vegetable
stock or equivalent in bouillon cubes,
dissolved in ½ cup boiling water

8 to 10 cups water, depending on
desired consistency

Salt and freshly ground black pepper to
taste

Potato chips, for serving

In a small frying pan, heat the olive oil over medium-high heat. Add the onion and tarragon and
sauté for 5 to 10 minutes, until the onions are translucent.

In a large soup pot, place the sautéed onions, nettle leaves, potato, and stock, add the water,
bring to a boil over high heat, and cook for 20 to 30 minutes, until the potatoes are soft.

Place the soup in the bowl of a food processor and blend (or use an immersion blender). Season
with salt and pepper to taste. Ladle the soup into individual bowls and garnish with a few potato
chips.

SERVES 10 TO 12

Sweet Potato and Corn Bisque

Here is a sweet and savory, cruelty-free, fishless bisque.

8 tablespoons (1 stick) vegan margarine

1 onion, diced

1 clove garlic, chopped

1 leek (white and light green parts only), sliced

½ cup dry white wine (optional)

1 tablespoon dried thyme

8 cups water

3 tablespoons powdered vegetable stock, or equivalent in bouillon cubes, dissolved in ½ cup boiling water

4 large sweet potatoes, chopped

One 8-ounce can corn, with liquid

Salt and freshly ground black pepper to taste

In a medium frying pan, melt the margarine over medium-high heat. Add the onion, garlic, and leek and sauté for 5 to 10 minutes, until the onions are translucent. Add the wine, if using, and the thyme and mix well.

In a large soup pot, bring the water to a boil over high heat. Add the stock, sweet potatoes, corn, and sautéed onion mixture. Bring the soup to a boil, reduce the heat to low, and simmer, covered, for about 30 minutes, until the potatoes are soft.

Place the soup in the bowl of a food processor and process (or use an immersion blender). Add more water if necessary to achieve the desired consistency. Season with salt and pepper to taste.

SERVES 8 TO 10

CREAMY SOUPS

These soups are not blended, but red lentils, potatoes, or other ingredients yield a creamy, smooth, gravy-like consistency.

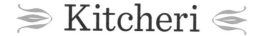

Kitcheri

In India, many yogis live on kitcheri only, which is a traditional ayurvedic healing food.

2 cups red lentils

1 cup short-grain brown rice or
    white basmati rice

8 cups water

1 tablespoon salt

In a large soup pot, place the lentils and rice, rinse with cold water, then drain. Add the water, bring to a boil over high heat, and cook for 5 minutes. Reduce the heat to medium-low and cook, covered, for an additional 45 minutes to 1 hour, stirring occasionally, until the lentils are dissolved and the rice is tender. Add more water if necessary to create a porridge-like consistency. Add the salt and stir well.

SERVES 8 TO 10

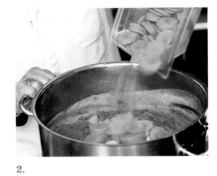

1.

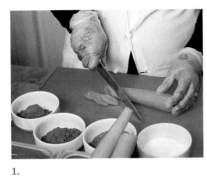

2.

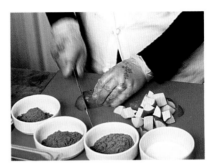

3.

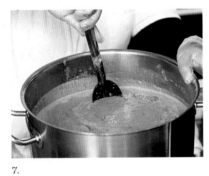

4.

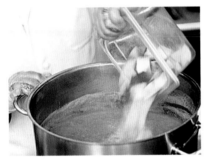

5.

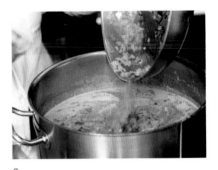

6.

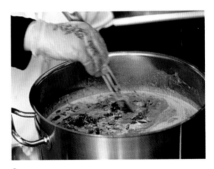

7.

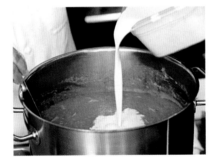

8.

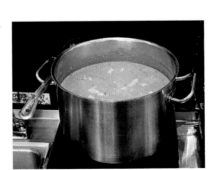

9.

10.

Maharini Dal

This classic Indian dal is fit for a queen, or maharini.
The secret is to sauté the dry spices before adding them to the pot.

2 cups red lentils

1 carrot, peeled and chopped

1 potato, unpeeled and diced

8 cups water, plus more as needed

⅓ cup vegetable oil, plus more as
    needed

1 onion, chopped

4 cloves garlic, chopped

1 tablespoon ground cumin

1 tablespoon ground coriander

1 tablespoon curry powder

½ bunch fresh cilantro, finely chopped

One 10- to 15-ounce can coconut milk

Salt and freshly ground black pepper to
    taste

In a large soup pot, place the lentils, rinse with cold water, then drain. Add the carrot, potato, and water to the pot and bring to a boil over high heat.

While the soup is heating, in a small frying pan, heat the vegetable oil over medium-high heat. Add the onion and garlic and sauté for 5 to 10 minutes, until the onions are translucent. In a small cup, mix the cumin, coriander, and curry powder with a little boiling water to dissolve, then add the spice mixture to the frying pan and sauté for another 1 to 2 minutes, adding a bit more oil or water to prevent the spices from burning.

When the soup is boiling, reduce the heat to medium-low and skim off any foam from the top. Add the sautéed mixture to the pot and cook, partially covered, for 1 hour. Stir in the cilantro, coconut milk, and salt and pepper to taste.

SERVES 10 TO 12

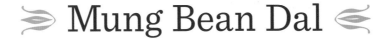 Mung Bean Dal

Mung beans give a fresh, green taste to the dal. Try ladling the soup over a large
spoonful of white or brown basmati rice and topping it with tofu sour cream.

2 cups mung beans

8¼ cups water

3 carrots, peeled and chopped into
small pieces

3 tablespoons sesame oil

½ red onion, chopped

6 cloves garlic, finely chopped

One 1-inch piece fresh ginger, peeled
and finely chopped

1 teaspoon ground cumin

1 tablespoon curry powder

1 teaspoon red pepper flakes

1 bunch fresh cilantro, leaves and stems
chopped

Salt to taste

In a large soup pot, place the mung beans and rinse with cold water, then drain. Add 8 cups of
the water, bring to a boil over high heat, then reduce the heat to medium-low and cook, partially
covered, for 1 hour, until soft. Add the carrots and raise the heat to medium.

While the carrots are cooking, in a small frying pan, heat the sesame oil over medium heat.
Add the onion, garlic, ginger, cumin, curry powder, and red pepper flakes and sauté for 3 minutes,
stirring often. Add the remaining ¼ cup water to the frying pan and simmer over low heat for
5 minutes.

Add the spice mixture and cilantro to the soup pot and stir well. Season with salt to taste.

SERVES 10 TO 12

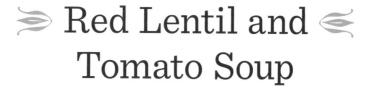 Red Lentil and Tomato Soup

The addition of tomatoes adds color and zest.

1 cup red lentils

8 cups water, plus more as needed

2 tablespoons vegetable oil

1 large onion, diced

1 tablespoon powdered vegetable stock
 or equivalent in bouillon cubes,
 dissolved in ¼ cup boiling water

1 teaspoon ground cumin

1 teaspoon curry powder

One 22-ounce can whole tomatoes or
 tomato sauce, or 2 pounds fresh
 tomatoes

1 cup coconut milk, soy milk, or almond
 milk

Salt and freshly ground black pepper to
 taste

In a large soup pot, place the lentils and rinse with cold water, then drain. Add the water and bring to a boil over high heat. Reduce the heat to medium-low and cook, partially covered, for about 45 minutes, until the lentils are mostly dissolved.

Meanwhile, in a small frying pan, heat the vegetable oil over medium-high heat. Add the onion and sauté for 5 to 10 minutes, until translucent. Add the stock, cumin, and curry powder and simmer for 3 minutes, stirring often and adding water if necessary to reach the consistency of a thin paste.

In the bowl of a food processor or blender, puree the tomatoes and coconut milk. Add the sautéed onion mixture and blend until smooth.

When the lentils are cooked, add the tomato mixture and more water as needed to obtain the desired consistency. Raise the heat to high and bring to a boil. Add salt and pepper to taste and remove from the heat.

SERVES 10 TO 12

Spicy Red Pepper– Lentil Soup

Bell peppers and jalapeños kindle a sweet fire.

1 cup red lentils

8 cups water

2 tablespoons tomato paste

½ cup fresh parsley, finely chopped

2 tablespoons powdered vegetable
stock or equivalent in bouillon cubes,
dissolved in ½ cup boiling water

1 red bell pepper

3 tablespoons olive oil

1 onion, chopped

1 fresh jalapeño pepper, chopped

1 tablespoon whole cumin seeds

1 tablespoon curry powder

Salt and freshly ground black pepper to
taste

In a large soup pot, place the lentils and rinse with cold water, then drain. Add the water and bring to a boil over high heat. Add the tomato paste, parsley, and stock and boil for 3 minutes. Reduce the heat to low and cook, partially covered, for about 45 minutes, until the lentils are mostly dissolved. Using an immersion blender, blend well.

While the lentils are cooking, roast the bell pepper over an open flame or broil it, turning it often, until it is charred all over, about 10 minutes. When cool enough to handle, remove and discard the stem and seeds, and cut the bell pepper into small pieces.

In a medium frying pan, heat the olive oil over medium-high heat. Add the onion, jalapeño, and cumin seeds and sauté, stirring often, for 5 to 10 minutes, until the onions are translucent. Add the chopped bell pepper and curry powder and mix, adding water as needed to form a sauce-like consistency. Reduce the heat to low and simmer for 3 minutes, then add to the blended lentils. Cook over low heat for about 5 minutes, then add salt and pepper to taste.

SERVES 8 TO 10

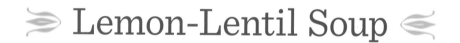 Lemon-Lentil Soup

This soup is light and lemony with a touch of spice. Add a little
chopped fresh ginger for an extra-invigorating rendition.

2 cups red lentils

10 cups water

2 tablespoons vegetable oil

3 cloves garlic, chopped

1 tablespoon ground cumin

1 tablespoon ground coriander

1 tablespoon curry powder

1 tablespoon salt

2 lemons, 1 juiced and 1 cut into 10 to
   12 thin slices (for serving)

2 cups cooked white basmati rice

½ bunch fresh cilantro, finely chopped

In a large soup pot, place the lentils and rinse with cold water, then drain. Add the water and bring to a boil over high heat, then reduce the heat to medium-low and simmer, partially covered, for about 45 minutes, until the lentils are mostly dissolved.

Meanwhile, in a small frying pan, heat the vegetable oil over medium heat. Add the garlic, cumin, coriander, and curry powder and sauté for 3 minutes, adding water as needed to make a thin paste. Add the sautéed garlic mixture to the soup. Just before serving, add the salt and lemon juice. Place a spoonful of rice into each serving bowl, then ladle the soup over the rice, float a lemon slice on top, and add a sprinkle of cilantro.

SERVES 10 TO 12

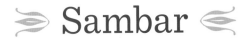 Sambar

This is a classic South Indian soup. Sambar powder is a spice blend that can be found in Indian grocery stores or online, as can hing and curry leaves.

½ cup red lentils

2 medium potatoes, peeled and diced into ½-inch pieces (about 2½ cups)

2½ cups peeled and diced butternut squash (½-inch pieces)

6 okra, sliced into ½-inch pieces

8 cups water

1½ tablespoons vegetable oil

2½ tablespoons sambar powder

1 cup diced tomatoes

1 tablespoon tomato paste

1 tablespoon tamarind paste

1 teaspoon salt, plus more to taste

Pinch of hing (also called asafoetida)

1 teaspoon mustard seeds

10 curry leaves

¼ cup chopped fresh cilantro

In a large soup pot, place the lentils and rinse with cold water, then drain. Add the potatoes, squash, okra, and water and bring to a boil over high heat. Reduce the heat to low and simmer, partially covered, for 30 minutes.

In a small frying pan, heat 1 tablespoon of the vegetable oil over medium-high heat. Add the sambar powder and sauté, stirring continuously, for 30 seconds, until well combined and fragrant.

Add the sautéed sambar powder, tomatoes, tomato paste, tamarind paste, salt, and hing to the soup pot and bring back to a boil over high heat. Reduce the heat to medium and simmer, covered, for 10 minutes.

Meanwhile, in a small frying pan, heat the remaining ½ tablespoon of oil and fry the mustard seeds, covered, for about 1 minute, until they pop, taking care not to let them burn. Add the mustard seeds, curry leaves, and cilantro to the soup pot and stir well. Add additional salt to taste.

SERVES 8 TO 10

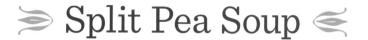 Split Pea Soup

This is one of the easiest soups to make and the most satisfying to eat.

2 cups dried split peas

2 carrots, peeled and cut into small
  pieces

8 cups water

Salt to taste

In a large soup pot, place the peas, cover with cold water by at least 4 inches, and let soak for at least 6 hours or overnight.

Rinse the peas with cold water and drain. Add the carrots and the water to the peas and bring to a boil over high heat. Boil for 5 minutes, reduce the heat to medium-low, and cook, partially covered, for 2 hours, stirring often, adding more water if necessary. Season with salt to taste and stir well.

SERVES 8 TO 10

Cauliflower-Curry Soup

Adding the cauliflower at the end leaves the flavors distinct. This soup is nice ladled over a large spoonful of white or brown basmati rice.

2 cups red lentils

3 carrots, peeled and chopped

3 potatoes, peeled and chopped

½ bunch fresh parsley, leaves and stems finely chopped

10 cups water

3 tablespoons vegetable oil

1 onion, chopped

6 cloves garlic, chopped

One 2-inch piece fresh ginger, peeled and finely chopped

1 teaspoon red pepper flakes

2 tablespoons tamarind paste

1 tablespoon ground cumin

1 tablespoon turmeric powder

1 tablespoon curry powder

1 head cauliflower, chopped into florets and lightly steamed

Two 10- to 15-ounce cans coconut milk

1 bunch fresh cilantro, leaves and stems finely chopped

1 tablespoon salt

In a large soup pot, place the lentils and rinse with cold water, then drain. Add the carrots, potatoes, parsley, and water and bring to a boil over high heat. Reduce the heat to medium-low and cook, covered, for 1 hour.

Meanwhile, in a small frying pan, heat the vegetable oil over medium-high heat. Add the onion, garlic, ginger, and red pepper flakes and sauté for 5 to 10 minutes, until the onions are translucent. Dissolve the tamarind paste, cumin, turmeric, and curry powder in a small amount of hot water, then add to the sauté pan, reduce the heat to low, and simmer for 5 minutes.

Add the sautéed onion mixture, cauliflower, coconut milk, cilantro, and salt to the soup pot and stir well.

SERVES 12 TO 14

French Tarragon Vegetable Soup

The licorice-like flavor of tarragon adds romance to the table, *oui*?

1 cup red lentils

2 medium potatoes, unpeeled and
   chopped into small pieces

½ head white cabbage, finely chopped

5 stalks celery with leaves, chopped

1 carrot, peeled and chopped

4 ounces frozen or canned corn

10 cups water

2 tablespoons olive oil

4 large cloves garlic, chopped

½ pound mushrooms, any variety, sliced

2 tablespoons dried tarragon

Salt and freshly ground black pepper to
   taste

Soy sauce, tamari, or Braggs Liquid
   Aminos to taste

In a large soup pot, place the lentils and rinse with cold water, then drain. Add the potatoes, cabbage, celery, carrot, corn, and water and bring to a boil over high heat. Reduce the heat to medium-low and simmer, partially covered, for about 45 minutes, until the vegetables are soft.

Meanwhile, in a medium frying pan, heat the olive oil over medium-high heat. Add the garlic, mushrooms, and tarragon and sauté for about 5 minutes, until the mushrooms are soft. Add the sautéed garlic mixture to the soup pot. Add salt, pepper, and soy sauce to taste.

SERVES 8 TO 10

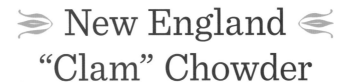 New England "Clam" Chowder

The chewy texture of the mushrooms and the sea-salty taste
of the kelp will fool any New England fisherman.

2 tablespoons olive oil

2 large potatoes, peeled (skin diced
and reserved) and cubed

Pinch of salt, plus more to taste

½ teaspoon vegan liquid smoke

1 medium onion, chopped

1 cup coarsely chopped shiitake or
oyster mushrooms

2 stalks celery, chopped

½ teaspoon dried thyme

1 teaspoon kelp granules or powder

3 tablespoons powdered vegetable
stock or equivalent in bouillon cubes,
dissolved in ½ cup boiling water

4 cups water

2 cups soy milk or almond milk

2 tablespoons fresh parsley, chopped

Freshly ground black pepper to taste

In a large saucepan, heat the olive oil over medium-high heat. Add the diced potato peels, salt,
and liquid smoke and sauté for 3 minutes, stirring frequently to avoid sticking. Add the onion and
mushrooms and cook, stirring frequently, for 5 to 10 minutes, until the onions are slightly soft-
ened. Add the potatoes, celery, thyme, kelp, stock, water, and soy milk. Reduce the heat to low and
simmer, covered, for about 25 minutes, stirring occasionally, until the potatoes are tender but not
falling apart. Add an additional cup of water or broth if you prefer a thinner consistency. Add the
parsley and salt and pepper to taste.

SERVES 6 TO 8

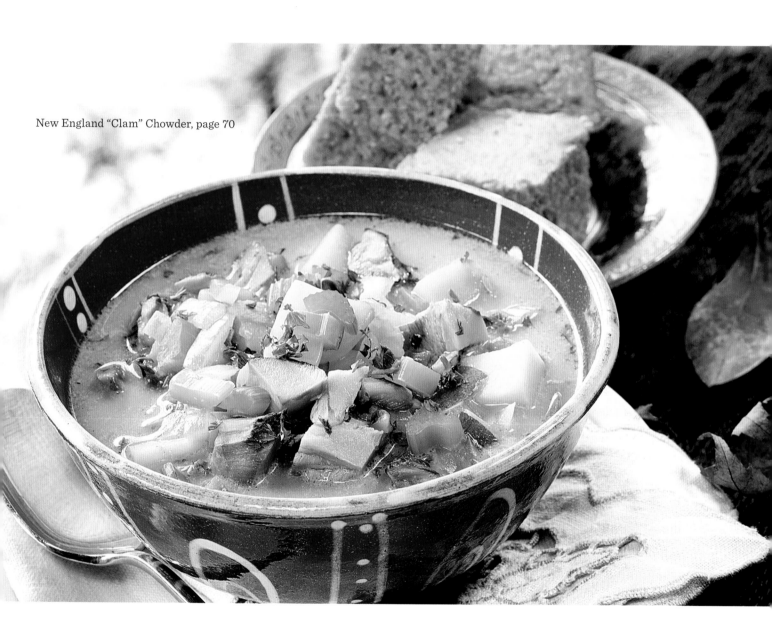

New England "Clam" Chowder, page 70

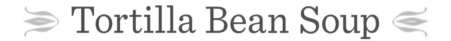 Tortilla Bean Soup

An easy twist on traditional Mexican fare,
this soup is just a can opener and a bag of chips away.

One 16-ounce can refried beans

One 8-inch corn tortilla, torn into small
pieces (or a handful of corn chips)

1 tablespoon powdered vegetable stock
or equivalent in bouillon cubes,
dissolved in ¼ cup boiling water

4 cups water

Corn chips (optional), for serving

In a medium soup pot, place the beans, tortilla, stock, and water, and bring to a boil over high heat, stirring well. Remove from the heat. Ladle the soup into individual bowls and garnish with a few corn chips if desired.

SERVES 2 TO 4

CHUNKY SOUPS

Chunks of vegetables in broth make a hearty stew.

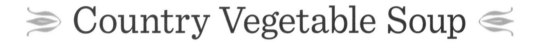

Country Vegetable Soup

The onions and herbs give this soup a distinctive country flavor.

2 medium Yellow Finn potatoes,
  unpeeled and chopped into small
  pieces
3 medium carrots, peeled and chopped
2 tablespoons powdered vegetable
  stock or equivalent in bouillon cubes,
  dissolved in ½ cup boiling water
10½ cups water
4 to 6 ounces frozen or canned corn
4 ounces frozen green peas

2 bay leaves
⅓ cup olive oil
2 medium yellow onions, chopped
6 cloves garlic, finely chopped
2 tablespoons dried rosemary
1 tablespoon ground coriander
1 tablespoon ground cumin
Salt and freshly ground black pepper to
  taste

In a large soup pot, place the potatoes, carrots, stock, and 10 cups of the water and bring to a boil over high heat. Reduce the heat to medium and cook, covered, for 20 minutes. Add the corn, peas, and bay leaves, reduce the heat to low, and cook, covered, for about 10 more minutes, until the potatoes are soft. Meanwhile, in a medium frying pan, heat the olive oil over medium-high heat. Add the onions, garlic, and rosemary and sauté for 3 minutes, stirring often. While the vegetables are sautéing, in a small bowl, combine the coriander and cumin. Add the remaining ½ cup water and mix to dissolve. Add the spiced water to the frying pan and simmer, covered, for 5 minutes. Add the sautéed onion mixture to the soup pot and simmer over medium-low heat for 5 minutes.

Add salt and pepper to taste. Discard the bay leaves.

SERVES 8 TO 10

⪜ Minestrone Soup ⪜

Minestrone is a thick Italian vegetable soup. The recipe is not fixed and can vary according to which vegetables are in season or on hand. Onions, tomatoes, carrots, and beans most often provide the base, usually with the addition of pasta, potatoes, or rice to add heartiness. I've provided a fairly simple recipe. Once mastered, feel free to improvise: add or delete according to your taste.

2 tablespoons olive oil

1 large red onion, chopped

4 button mushrooms, thinly sliced

1 large carrot, peeled and diced into small pieces

1 medium zucchini, diced into small pieces

1 teaspoon dried thyme

1 teaspoon dried oregano

1 teaspoon dried basil

One 15-ounce can red kidney beans, with their liquid

One 28-ounce can diced tomatoes, with their juices

3 tablespoons powdered vegetable stock or equivalent in bouillon cubes, dissolved in ½ cup boiling water

8 cups water

1 cup dry penne rigate pasta, elbow macaroni, or any type of small pasta

½ cup frozen cut green beans

½ cup frozen green peas

4 sprigs fresh parsley, finely chopped

½ cup kale or spinach, chopped into small pieces

1 teaspoon salt, plus more to taste

¼ teaspoon freshly ground black pepper, plus more to taste

In a large soup pot, heat the olive oil over medium-high heat. Add the onion and sauté for 5 to 10 minutes, until translucent. Add the mushrooms, carrot, zucchini, thyme, oregano, and basil and cook for about 5 minutes, until the carrots soften. Add the kidney beans with their liquid, tomatoes with their juices, stock, and water and bring to a boil over high heat. Add the pasta, green beans, and peas and cook for 7 to 10 minutes, until the pasta is tender. Add the parsley, kale, salt, and pepper. Taste the soup and add more salt and pepper as needed.

SERVES 6 TO 8

Hearty Vegetable Soup

Here is a warm and comforting soup, especially on a cold day.

½ cup barley

12 cups water

1 yam, peeled and cut into small pieces

2 red potatoes, peeled and cut into
small pieces

2 large beets, peeled and cut into small
pieces

6 stalks celery, cut into small pieces

1 cup finely shredded red cabbage

10 fresh green beans, cut into small
pieces

½ cup frozen or canned corn

One 15-ounce can red kidney beans,
with their liquid

¼ cup dried nori seaweed, cut into small
pieces

2 bay leaves

⅓ cup olive oil

6 cloves garlic, finely chopped

1 onion, finely chopped

4 sprigs fresh parsley, finely chopped

1 teaspoon dried thyme

1 teaspoon dried basil

1 teaspoon dried oregano

2 tablespoons powdered vegetable
stock or equivalent in bouillon cubes,
dissolved in ½ cup boiling water

Salt and freshly ground black pepper to
taste

In a large soup pot, place the barley and rinse with cold water, then drain. Add the water and bring to a boil over high heat. Reduce the heat to low and cook, covered, for about 10 minutes, until the barley is beginning to expand. Add the yam, potatoes, beets, celery, cabbage, green beans, corn, kidney beans, seaweed, and bay leaves. Raise the heat to medium-low and cook, covered, for about 30 minutes, until the potatoes are soft.

Meanwhile, in a medium frying pan, heat the olive oil over medium-high heat. Add the garlic and onion, and sauté for 5 to 10 minutes, until the onions are translucent. Add the parsley, thyme, basil, and oregano and cook for 3 more minutes.

Add the sautéed garlic mixture and the stock to the soup pot and cook, covered, for an additional 10 minutes. Discard the bay leaves. Add salt and pepper to taste.

SERVES 10 TO 12

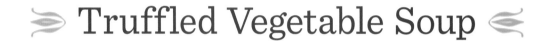 Truffled Vegetable Soup

Truffle oil elevates a simple soup to five-star dining. White truffle oil tends to have a stronger flavor than black and I prefer it, but if it is not available, go with what you can get.

2 medium potatoes, peeled and cut into small cubes

1 zucchini, cut into small, thin slices

2 carrots, peeled and cut into small, thin slices

½ cup fresh or frozen green peas

6 baby portabella mushrooms, sliced very thin

3 tablespoons powdered vegetable stock or equivalent in bouillon cubes, dissolved in ½ cup boiling water

1 tablespoon onion powder

1 teaspoon garlic powder

1 teaspoon dried sage

1 teaspoon dried tarragon

1 teaspoon herbes de Provence

8 cups water

1 cup almond milk or soy milk

Salt and freshly ground black pepper to taste

Truffle oil, for serving

In a large soup pot, place the potatoes, zucchini, carrots, peas, mushrooms, stock, onion powder, garlic powder, sage, tarragon, herbes de Provence, and water and bring to a boil over high heat. Reduce the heat to low, cover, and simmer for 20 to 30 minutes, until the vegetables are soft. Add the almond milk and simmer for 1 more minute. Add salt and pepper to taste. Ladle the soup into individual bowls and garnish with 1 or 2 drops of truffle oil.

SERVES 8 TO 10

⇌ Asian-Style ⇌ Seaweed-Vegetable Soup

This soup is a meal in itself.

6 dried shiitake mushrooms

2 tablespoons powdered vegetable
   stock or equivalent in bouillon cubes,
   dissolved in ½ cup boiling water

½ cup dried wakame seaweed

8 cups water

1 scallion, chopped into small pieces

2 stalks celery, finely chopped

2 leaves bok choy, cut into small pieces

4 leaves napa cabbage, cut into small
   pieces

1 cup spinach leaves, cut into small
   pieces

1 cup mung bean sprouts

4 ounces firm tofu, cut into small cubes

Toasted sesame oil, for serving

3 sprigs fresh cilantro, finely chopped,
   for serving

Soy sauce, tamari, or Braggs Liquid
   Aminos to taste

In a small bowl, place the mushrooms, add boiling water to cover, and let stand for 5 to 10 minutes to rehydrate.

Meanwhile, place the stock, seaweed, and water in a large soup pot and bring to a boil over high heat. When the mushrooms are soft, drain the soaking water into the soup pot. Cut the mushrooms into thin strips and add them to the pot along with the scallions. Return the soup to a boil and boil for 5 minutes. Add the celery, bok choy, cabbage, spinach, sprouts, and tofu and cook for 3 minutes (do not overcook). Ladle the soup into individual bowls, garnish with several drops of sesame oil, sprinkle with cilantro, sprinkle with serve with soy sauce to taste.

SERVES 8 TO 10

Potato, Bean, and Barley Soup

Don't let the number of ingredients fool you—this soup is extremely easy to prepare.

2 tablespoons olive oil

1 medium onion, chopped

Cloves from 1 whole garlic bulb, finely chopped

1 tablespoon dried rosemary

4 large russet potatoes, peeled and chopped into small pieces

One 12-ounce can navy beans

½ cup pearl barley

3 carrots, peeled and chopped into small pieces

¼ pound fresh green beans, chopped into 1-inch pieces

4 ounces frozen corn

6 ounces fresh or frozen green peas

3 bay leaves

1 tablespoon ground cumin

1 teaspoon ground coriander

1 teaspoon dried sage

10 cups water

2 teaspoons salt

½ teaspoon freshly ground black pepper

In a large soup pot, heat the olive oil over medium-high heat. Add the onion, garlic, and rosemary and sauté for 5 to 10 minutes, until the onions are translucent. Add the potatoes, beans, barley, carrots, string beans, corn, peas, bay leaves, cumin, coriander, sage, and water and bring to a rapid boil over high heat. Reduce the heat to medium-low and cook for 1 hour. Discard the bay leaves. Add the salt and pepper.

SERVES 10 TO 12

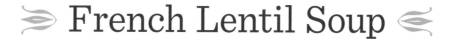 French Lentil Soup

Here is a French country stew.

4 cups French lentils

2 tablespoons vegetable oil

6 cloves garlic, finely chopped

6 scallions, finely chopped

3 potatoes, peeled and chopped into
  small pieces

3 carrots, peeled and chopped into
  small pieces

1 tablespoon herbes de Provence

10 cups water

Salt to taste

In a large soup pot, place the lentils and rinse with cold water, then drain.

In a small frying pan, heat the vegetable oil over medium heat. Add the garlic and onions and sauté for 5 to 10 minutes, until the scallions are translucent.

Add the sautéed garlic mixture, potatoes, carrots, herbes de Provence, and water to the soup pot and bring to a boil over high heat. Reduce the heat to medium and cook, covered, for 1 hour. Season with salt to taste.

SERVES 8 TO 10

⇌ White Bean and Kale Soup ⇌

The kale adds both color and calcium.

1 large white or yellow onion, finely
    chopped
One 1-inch strip kombu seaweed, cut
    into small pieces
2 tablespoons powdered vegetable
    stock or equivalent in bouillon cubes,
    dissolved in ½ cup boiling water
2 teaspoons dried oregano
2 teaspoons dried rosemary
1 teaspoon dried sage

1 teaspoon onion powder
1 teaspoon garlic powder
8 cups water
Two 15-ounce cans cannellini beans,
    with their liquid
2 cups loosely packed finely chopped
    kale
Salt and freshly ground black pepper to
    taste

In a large soup pot, place the onion, kombu, stock, oregano, rosemary, sage, onion powder, garlic powder, and water and bring to a boil over high heat. Reduce the heat to low and cook, covered, for 15 minutes.

Place 1 can of the beans with their liquid in the bowl of a food processor and process until smooth (or place the beans in a large bowl and blend using an immersion blender). Add the blended beans and the remaining can of beans with their liquid to the soup pot. Add the kale and cook, covered, for another 10 minutes. Add salt and pepper to taste.

SERVES 8 TO 10

Savory Pumpkin Soup

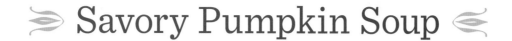

I've been told this classy soup tastes like it should be on the menu
of the fanciest restaurants in the world.

2 tablespoons (¼ stick) vegan
   margarine

1 large red or yellow onion, finely
   chopped

1 cup scallions, finely chopped

2 tablespoons powdered vegetable
   stock or equivalent in bouillon cubes,
   dissolved in ½ cup boiling water

One 15-ounce can pureed pumpkin

2 teaspoons maple syrup

1 bay leaf

½ cup finely chopped fresh parsley

2 teaspoons curry powder

½ teaspoon ground nutmeg

½ teaspoon ground coriander

½ teaspoon salt

½ teaspoon freshly ground black
   pepper

6 cups water

¼ cup almond milk or soy milk

1 tablespoon walnut oil

In a large soup pot, melt the margarine over medium-high heat. Add the onion and scallions and
sauté for 5 to 10 minutes, until the onions are translucent. Add the stock, pumpkin, maple syrup,
bay leaf, parsley, curry powder, nutmeg, coriander, salt, pepper, and water and bring to a boil over
high heat. Reduce the heat to low and simmer, uncovered, for 15 to 20 minutes, until the flavors
are well integrated. Discard the bay leaf. Stir in the almond milk and walnut oil.

SERVES 4 TO 6

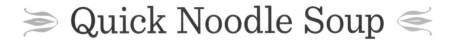 Quick Noodle Soup

I often make this soup for myself as a late-night pick-me-up,

and it takes less than ten minutes to prepare.

1 dried shiitake mushroom, broken into
    small pieces

1 teaspoon dried hijiki seaweed

1 tablespoon powdered vegetable stock
    or equivalent in bouillon cubes,
    dissolved in ¼ cup boiling water

2 cups water

1 ounce bean thread or rice noodles

¼ cup chopped greens (spinach, napa
    cabbage, bok choy, or other)

1 teaspoon toasted sesame oil

Soy sauce, tamari, or Braggs Liquid
    Aminos to taste

In a medium pot, place the mushroom, seaweed, stock, and water, bring to a boil over high heat, and boil for 3 minutes. Add the noodles and cook for 1 more minute, then turn off the heat. Add the chopped greens, sesame oil, and soy sauce to taste.

SERVES 1 TO 2

Simple Tahini-Shoyu Noodle Soup

The distinction of this soup is the broth, which is based on tahini and shoyu, the Japanese term for soy sauce.

4 ounces uncooked pasta (linguine, udon, soba, glass noodles, or rice noodles)

6 cups water

1 tablespoon tahini

2 tablespoons soy sauce, tamari, or Braggs Liquid Aminos

1 teaspoon dried hijiki seaweed

1 teaspoon powdered vegetable stock or equivalent in bouillon cubes, dissolved in ¼ cup boiling water

1 cup fresh spinach, chopped

Prepare the pasta according to the directions on the package, drain, and set aside.

Fill a large soup pot with the water and bring to a rapid boil. Meanwhile, in a small cup or bowl, mix the tahini and soy sauce to make a paste and set aside.

Place the seaweed in a small bowl and add boiling water to cover. Let stand for about 5 minutes, until the seaweed is rehydrated.

To the soup pot, add the stock, pasta, tahini mixture, rehydrated seaweed, and spinach. Stir to incorporate all of the ingredients.

SERVES 6 TO 8

⮜ Curry-Tahini-Shoyu ⮞ Noodle Soup

This is a mildly spicy Japanese country stew.

4 ounces uncooked noodles (udon, soba, glass noodles, or rice noodles)

1 sweet potato, peeled or unpeeled and chopped into small cubes

¼ pound fresh green beans, chopped into small pieces

1 medium carrot, peeled and chopped into small pieces

1 stalk celery, chopped into small pieces

6 ounces fresh, frozen, or canned corn

One 16-ounce can adzuki beans, with liquid

2 tablespoons powdered vegetable stock or equivalent in bouillon cubes, dissolved in ½ cup boiling water

3 tablespoons dried hijiki seaweed

8 cups water

2 tablespoons tahini

2 tablespoons mellow white miso

2 tablespoons vegetable oil

One 1-inch piece fresh ginger, peeled and finely chopped

3 cloves garlic, finely chopped

1 medium onion, chopped into small pieces

2 teaspoons curry powder

1 teaspoon ground coriander

1 teaspoon ground cumin

8 ounces firm tofu, chopped into small cubes

2 teaspoons salt

½ teaspoon freshly ground black pepper or cayenne pepper

Hot or toasted sesame oil, for serving

Prepare the noodles according to the directions on the package, drain, and set aside. In a large soup pot, place the sweet potato, green beans, carrot, celery, corn, beans, stock, seaweed, and water, and bring to a boil over high heat. Reduce the heat to medium-low and cook, covered, for about 20 minutes, until the vegetables are soft.

Meanwhile, in a small bowl, mix the tahini and miso to make a paste, then set aside.

In a small frying pan, heat the oil over medium heat. Add the ginger, garlic, and onion and sauté for 5 to 10 minutes, until the onions are translucent. Add the curry powder, coriander, and cumin and cook for about 3 minutes, adding just enough water to keep the mixture from burning, until well mixed and the spices are fragrant.

Add the noodles, sautéed mixture, tahini/miso mix, tofu, salt, and pepper to the pot. Stir gently to incorporate all of the ingredients. Ladle the soup into individual bowls and add several drops of sesame oil in each bowl.

SERVES 6 TO 8

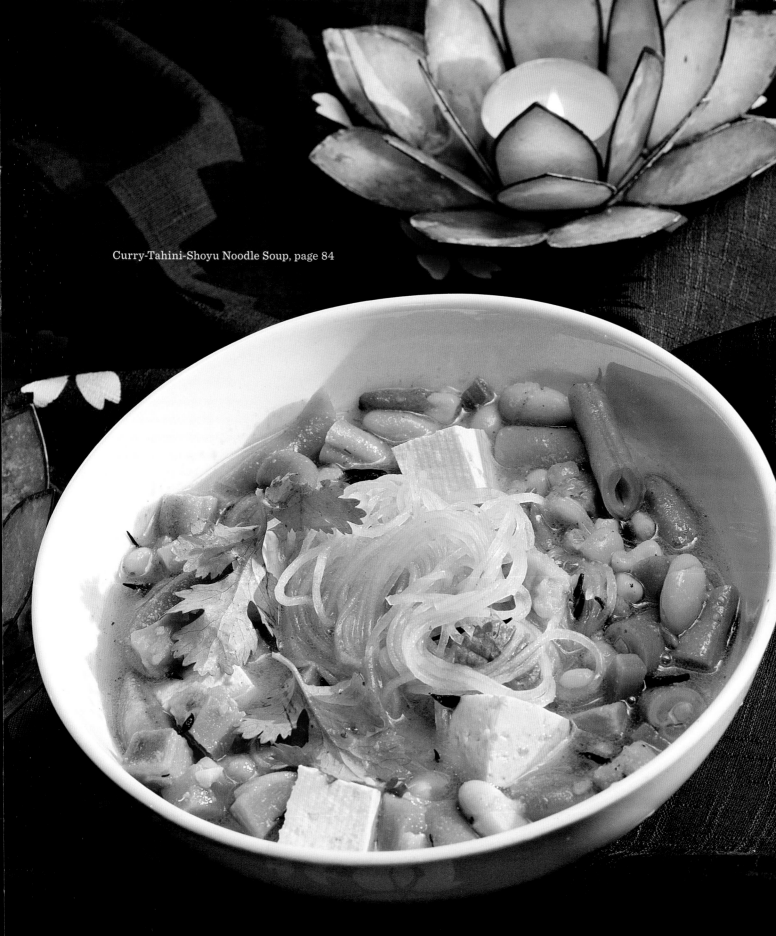

Curry-Tahini-Shoyu Noodle Soup, page 84

⋙ Pea Pod–Noodle Soup ⋘

This soup features fresh pea pods and tofu floating in a creamy coconut broth.

1 pound uncooked rice noodles or other
    noodles
6 cups water
3 tablespoons toasted sesame oil
One 1-inch piece fresh ginger, peeled
    and finely chopped
One 6- to 8-ounce block firm tofu, cut
    into small cubes
4 to 6 sun-dried tomatoes, sliced into
    thin strips

1 cup fresh pea pods
1 cup mung bean sprouts
½ cup fresh, frozen, or canned corn
    kernels
One 10- to 15-ounce can coconut milk
Hot sesame oil to taste
Red pepper flakes to taste
Soy sauce, tamari, Braggs Liquid
    Aminos, or salt to taste

Prepare the noodles according to the directions on the package, drain, and set aside.

Fill a large soup pot with the water and bring to a boil over high heat.

Meanwhile, in a large frying pan, heat the sesame oil over medium heat. Add the ginger, tofu, and tomatoes and sauté for 5 minutes.

Add the sautéed mixture, pea pods, sprouts, and corn to the pot, stir well, and add the coconut milk. Add the noodles and stir well. Ladle the soup into individual bowls and top with a few drops of hot sesame oil, a few red pepper flakes, and a few drops of soy sauce, all to taste.

SERVES 6 TO 8

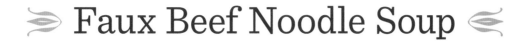 Faux Beef Noodle Soup

The mushrooms and hijiki give this soup a beef-like flavor,
and the seitan provides a beef-like texture.

5 dried shiitake mushrooms

½ cup dried hijiki seaweed

6 cups water

1 tablespoon powdered vegetable stock
 or equivalent in bouillon cubes,
 dissolved in ¼ cup boiling water

1 cup seitan, cut into bite-size pieces

3 ounces thin rice noodles

1 cup densely packed chopped spinach
 or arugula leaves

Salt and/or soy sauce, tamari, or Braggs
 Liquid Aminos to taste

Place the mushrooms and seaweed in a small bowl and add boiling water to cover. Let stand for 5 to 10 minutes to rehydrate.

Drain the soaking liquid into a large soup pot, reserving the mushrooms and seaweed. Add the water and the stock to the pot and bring to a boil over high heat.

Meanwhile, place the mushrooms and seaweed in the bowl of a food processor and chop fine (do not puree; retain a chunky consistency). Transfer the mushroom mixture to the soup pot and add the seitan. When the broth is at a full boil, add the noodles and cook for 2 to 3 minutes, until the noodles are soft and the ingredients are well combined. Just before serving, add the spinach and salt and/or soy sauce to taste.

SERVES 6 TO 8

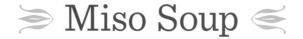 Miso Soup

Using chickpea miso makes this soup light and sweet. Because of the presence of delicate enzymes, miso soup should not be left in a pot on the stove for a prolonged period of time but rather prepared as individual servings.

1 teaspoon wakame seaweed

1 cup boiling water, plus more to
 rehydrate the seaweed

1 tablespoon chickpea miso

Four ¼-inch cubes cold, firm tofu

Cayenne pepper to taste

In a small bowl, place the seaweed and add boiling water to cover. Let stand for about 5 minutes to rehydrate.

Place the miso in a serving bowl and add 2 tablespoons of the boiling water; whisk until the miso is blended. Add the tofu, rehydrated seaweed, and the remaining ¾ cup plus 2 tablespoons boiling water to the bowl. Stir and serve immediately with a sprinkle of cayenne pepper to taste.

SERVES 1

Green Lemon-Ginger Soup

I tend to prefer savory to sweet, so opt for this soup over a glass of juice.

1 teaspoon spirulina powder

¼ teaspoon finely chopped fresh peeled ginger

1 tablespoon powdered vegetable stock or equivalent in bouillon cubes, dissolved in ¼ cup boiling water

Sprinkle of cayenne pepper

¼ teaspoon lemon juice

¼ teaspoon maple syrup

1 cup boiling water

Flaxseed oil, for serving

In a small bowl or cup, place the spirulina, ginger, stock, cayenne, lemon juice, maple syrup, and water. Stir well and top with a few drops of flaxseed oil.

SERVES 1

Clear and Light Savory Soup

This is a great lead-in to a hearty meal.

½ zucchini, chopped into small pieces

½ carrot, peeled and chopped into small pieces

4 to 6 fresh green beans, chopped into small pieces

3 baby portabella or button mushrooms, very thinly sliced

2 tablespoons powdered vegetable stock or equivalent in bouillon cubes, dissolved in ½ cup boiling water

1 teaspoon onion powder

1 teaspoon dried sage

1 teaspoon dried tarragon

1 teaspoon herbes de Provence

6 cups water

In a medium saucepan, place the zucchini, carrot, green beans, mushrooms, stock, onion powder, sage, tarragon, herbes de Provence, and water and bring to a boil over high heat. Reduce the heat to low and cook, covered, for about 25 minutes, until the vegetables are soft.

SERVES 4 TO 6

RAW SOUPS

Raw soups are very much like blended salads or smoothies.
They are satisfying and easily digested, much like green juice,
but retain more fiber. I offer seven varieties here,
but don't hold back—be creative!

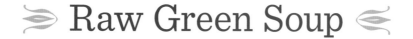 Raw Green Soup

8 large leaves romaine lettuce

1 stalk celery, coarsely chopped

1 leaf kale

½ cucumber, peeled and coarsely
   chopped

4 cherry tomatoes

1 tablespoon olive oil

1 tablespoon lemon juice

Pinch of sea salt

1 to 2 cups water

In the bowl of a food processor or in a heavy-duty blender jar, place the lettuce, celery, kale, cucumber, tomatoes, olive oil, lemon juice, salt, and water and blend, adding enough water to yield a smooth and creamy consistency. Pour into a glass.

SERVES 1

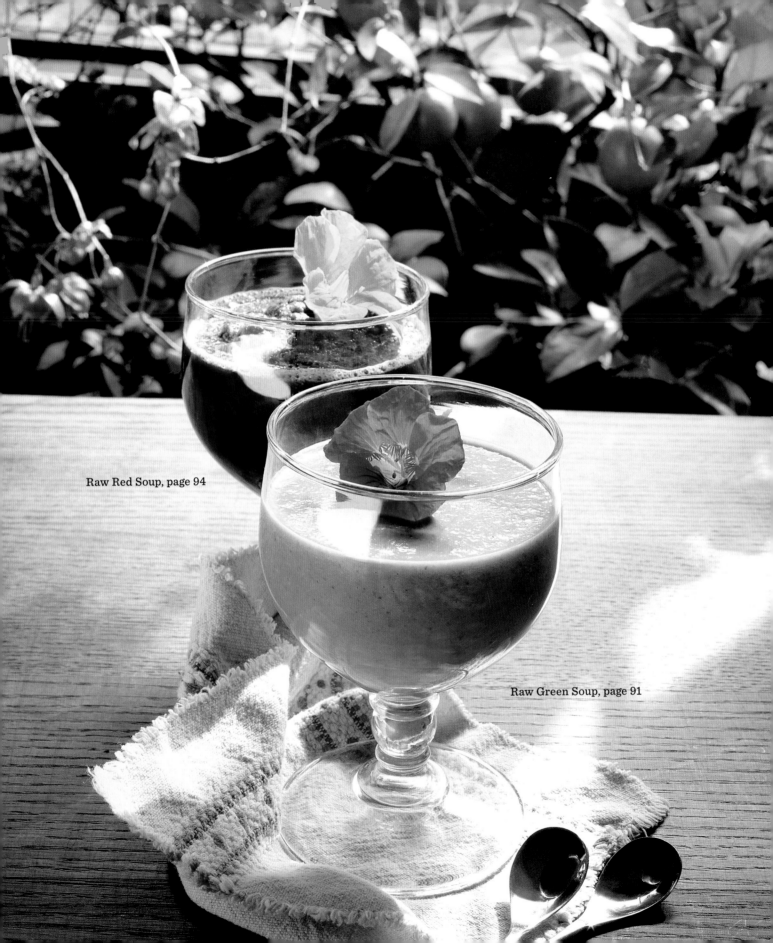

Raw Red Soup, page 94

Raw Green Soup, page 91

⋑ Very Green Raw Soup ⋐

2½ cups mixed lettuce greens,
  tightly packed
4 cherry tomatoes
½ apple, cored
1 teaspoon spirulina powder

1 tablespoon olive oil
1 teaspoon lemon juice
Salt and freshly ground black pepper to
  taste
1 to 2 cups water

In the bowl of a food processor or in a heavy-duty blender jar, place the lettuce, tomatoes, apple, spirulina, olive oil, lemon juice, salt and pepper to taste, and water and blend, adding enough water to yield a smooth and creamy consistency. Pour into a glass.

SERVES 1

⋑ Spinach-Avocado ⋐ Raw Soup

1 bunch spinach, as much as you would
  put in a salad
½ avocado
1 tablespoon lemon juice

1 tablespoon olive oil
Salt and freshly ground black pepper to
  taste
1 to 2 cups water

In the bowl of a food processor or in a heavy-duty blender jar, place the spinach, avocado, lemon juice, olive oil, salt and pepper to taste, and water, and blend, adding enough water to yield a smooth and creamy consistency. Pour into a glass.

SERVES 1

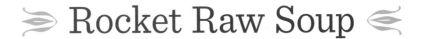 Rocket Raw Soup

1 bunch arugula

1 cucumber, peeled

½ apple, cored

1 tablespoon olive oil

1 teaspoon balsamic vinegar

1 to 2 cups water

In the bowl of a food processor or in a heavy-duty blender jar, place the arugula, cucumber, apple, olive oil, vinegar, and water and blend, adding just enough water to yield a smooth and creamy consistency. Pour into a glass.

SERVES 1

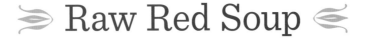 Raw Red Soup

1 apple, cored

1 beet, peeled and coarsely chopped

1 carrot, peeled and coarsely chopped

2 tablespoons lemon juice

1 to 2 cups water

In the bowl of a food processor or in a heavy-duty blender jar, place the apple, beet, carrot, lemon juice, and water and blend, adding enough water to yield a smooth and creamy consistency. Pour into a glass.

SERVES 1

Raw Shoots-Roots-Fruits Soup

½ apple, cored

½ carrot, peeled or unpeeled

½ beet, peeled and coarsely chopped

4 cherry tomatoes

1 tablespoon spirulina powder

1 tablespoon lemon juice

1 to 2 cups water

4 leaves red-leaf lettuce

4 leaves arugula

2 leaves dandelion greens

In the bowl of a food processor or in a heavy-duty blender jar, place the apple, carrot, beet, tomatoes, spirulina, lemon juice, and water and blend, adding enough water to yield a smooth and creamy consistency. Add the lettuce, arugula, and dandelion greens and blend until smooth. Pour into a glass.

SERVES 1

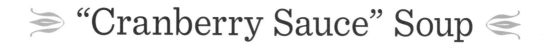 "Cranberry Sauce" Soup

1 carrot, peeled or unpeeled

1 beet, peeled and coarsely chopped

1 apple, cored

One ½-inch piece fresh ginger, peeled and coarsely chopped

1 tablespoon lemon juice

1 to 2 cups water

In the bowl of a food processor or in a heavy-duty blender jar, place the carrot, beet, apple, ginger, lemon juice and water and blend, adding enough water to yield a smooth and creamy consistency. Pour into a glass.

SERVES 1

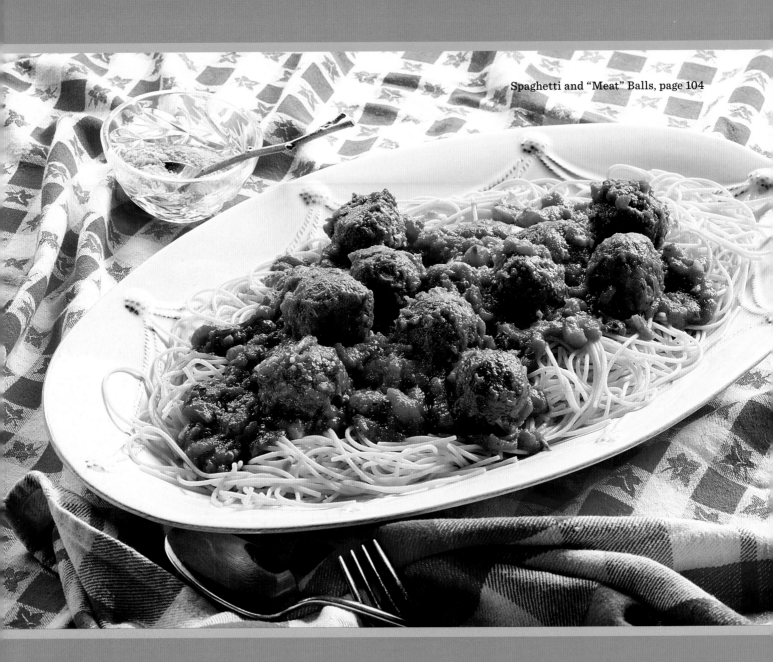

Spaghetti and "Meat" Balls, page 104

Pasta and Sauces

Pasta refers to noodles, which can be made from a variety of sources. The taste comes from not only the ingredients but also from the texture, which is derived in part from the shape of the noodles. Pasta can be made from the flour of many grains and vegetables, including wheat, rice, corn, millet, potatoes, green beans, and mung beans. Wheat pasta is the most popular in the West and comes in many shapes, from spaghetti and angel hair to penne and elbow macaroni. The variety of pasta and noodles in Asian cooking is more extensive and includes not only pasta made from different types of wheat but also naturally gluten-free varieties made from rice, buckwheat (soba), green beans, and mung beans. The pasta is fashioned into many different shapes, including fat threads, flat threads, long threads, and dumplings. Noodles made from green beans or mung beans are called saifun, cellophane, or glass noodles, because when cooked, they are clear and look like glass. Usually pasta and noodles are served or mixed with a sauce or seasoned with oil, herbs, or spices. A few of the pasta sauces in this chapter, like pesto, can be served over grains or potatoes or spread on bread or crackers.

⥸ Pasta with Pesto ⥺

Basil pesto is best eaten fresh, as the green color begins to blacken quickly. To prolong the freshness, sprinkle additional vitamin C powder (approximately ½ teaspoon) over the top of the sauce and store in the refrigerator. Pesto can also be frozen. And it's flexible: you can substitute walnuts or almonds for the pine nuts, and you can substitute parsley or arugula for the basil. Lots of wild mustard grows like a weed on the grounds of the Wild Woodstock Jivamukti Forest Sanctuary in Woodstock, New York, and in the spring and early summer I make pesto using wild mustard instead of basil. If wild mustard is available to you, use this same basic recipe but leave out the garlic cloves and ascorbic acid—you won't need them. I like to use rotini pasta for pesto because the spiral shape of the pasta holds the pesto better.

4 cups densely packed fresh basil leaves

½ cup pine nuts

½ cup olive oil

1½ tablespoons brown rice miso, or use mellow white miso for milder pesto

2 tablespoons lemon juice

2 tablespoons nutritional yeast flakes

2 cloves garlic (optional)

¼ teaspoon vitamin C powder (pure ascorbic acid, with no buffers)

½ teaspoon freshly ground black pepper

1 pound uncooked rotini pasta

In the bowl of a food processor, place the basil, pine nuts, olive oil, miso, lemon juice, nutritional yeast, garlic, if using, vitamin C powder, and pepper and process. Do not overprocess—pesto is best when it is slightly chunky. Set aside.

Prepare the pasta according to the directions on the package, then drain. Stir the pesto into the pasta or plate the pasta and top with a large dollop of pesto.

SERVES 4 TO 6

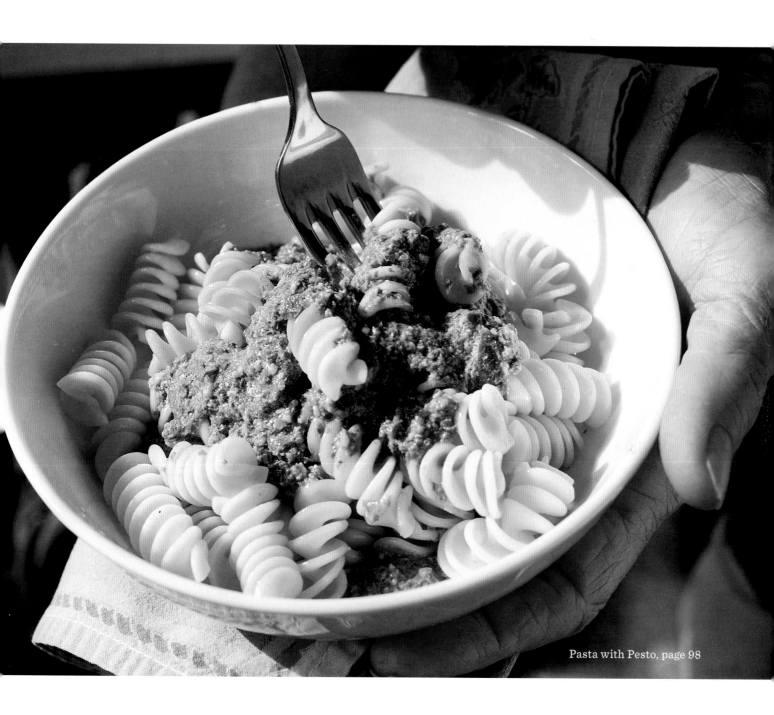

Pasta with Pesto, page 98

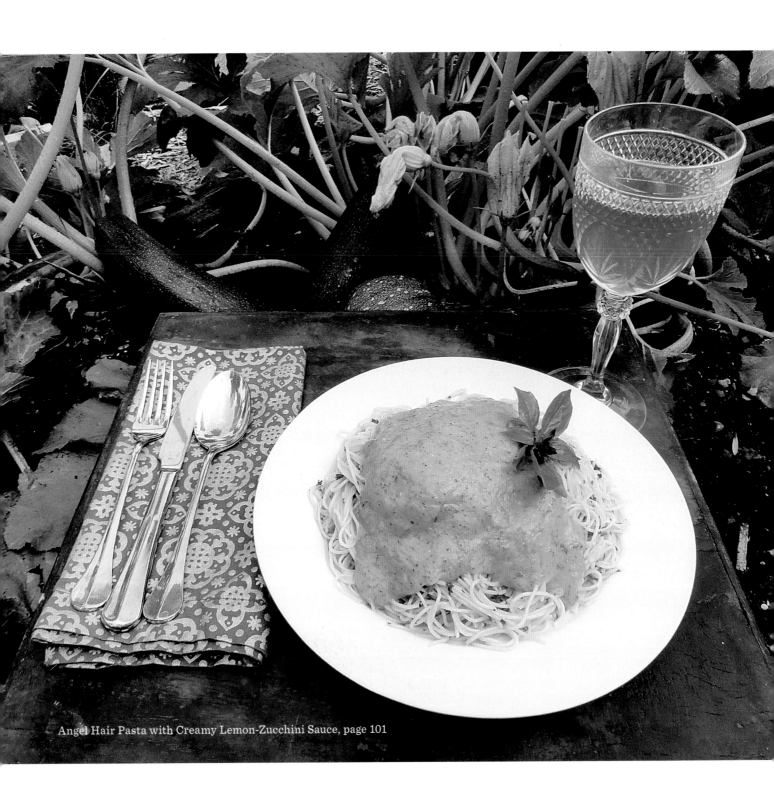

Angel Hair Pasta with Creamy Lemon-Zucchini Sauce, page 101

Angel Hair Pasta with Creamy Lemon-Zucchini Sauce

I like angel hair pasta for this recipe because its lightness complements the delicate nature of the sauce, but any type of pasta will work well. For a "corny" version, place ½ cup fresh or frozen corn kernels in the colander or strainer, then drain the pasta over the corn, transfer the mixture back into the pasta pot, and stir well. This sauce thickens as it cools and can be used as a light, creamy salad dressing, or warm it back up and serve it as an elegant soup garnished with parsley.

5 pounds zucchini (3 to 6 zucchini, depending on their size), sliced into ½-inch pieces

3 tablespoons lemon juice

½ cup coconut oil or 8 tablespoons (1 stick) vegan margarine

2 tablespoons dried tarragon

1 teaspoon salt

½ teaspoon freshly ground black pepper

1 pound uncooked angel hair pasta

In a steamer basket set over boiling water place the zucchini and steam for about 20 minutes, until soft.

Place the zucchini, lemon juice, coconut oil, tarragon, salt, and pepper in a food processor or blender and blend until smooth and creamy.

Prepare the pasta according to the directions on the package, then drain. Plate the pasta and top with a large dollop of sauce.

SERVES 4 TO 6

≈ Spaghetti All'aglio e Olio ≈

Spaghetti all'aglio e olio means "spaghetti with garlic and oil" in Italian. I have added some additional herbs to this popular, traditional recipe. But using a bit of the pasta cooking water is the secret ingredient of this dish. I learned this trick from Joe Sponzo and Rob Frabone, both incredible Italian chefs who told me that many restaurants in Italy prize pasta water like fine stock, and they will use the same water throughout the day to cook all of the pasta, topping it off occasionally as needed. This trick can be used for any of the Italian-style pasta recipes in this book.

One 8-ounce package uncooked
   spaghetti
½ cup olive oil
8 large cloves garlic, finely chopped
1 tablespoon dried oregano
1 teaspoon dried rosemary

1½ teaspoons red pepper flakes
⅓ cup chopped fresh parsley
Nutritional yeast flakes or commercially
   prepared vegan Parmesan cheese,
   for serving (optional)
Salt to taste

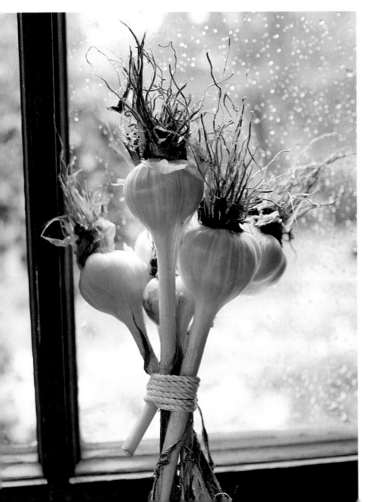

Prepare the pasta according to the directions on the package. Drain, but reserve ½ cup of the cooking water. Set aside.

In a deep frying pan, heat the olive oil over medium heat. Add the garlic, oregano, rosemary, and red pepper flakes and sauté for 2 to 3 minutes, stirring frequently to prevent the garlic from burning. Remove from the heat and add the pasta and the reserved pasta cooking water. Toss and stir so that the oil and water emulsify. Add the parsley and top with nutritional yeast, if desired, and salt to taste.

SERVES 2 TO 4

Pasta with Tomato Sauce

I experimented for years to come up with what I feel is the perfect basic tomato sauce.
It lends itself to any creative variation.

3 tablespoons olive oil

4 large cloves garlic, finely chopped

1 teaspoon dried rosemary

1 teaspoon dried oregano

10 leaves fresh basil, finely chopped or
    left whole, or 1 tablespoon dried basil

One 28-ounce can tomato puree, or
    1 pound fresh tomatoes pureed in the
    bowl of a food processor

1 teaspoon agave

1 teaspoon salt

¼ teaspoon red pepper flakes

1 pound uncooked pasta, any kind

Nutritional yeast flakes or commercially
    prepared vegan Parmesan cheese,
    for serving (optional)

In a deep frying pan or a large saucepan, heat the olive oil over medium heat. Add the garlic, rosemary, oregano, and basil and sauté for 2 minutes, stirring frequently to prevent the garlic from burning. Reduce the heat to low and add the tomato puree, agave, salt, and red pepper flakes. Simmer for 15 minutes, stirring often.

Prepare the pasta according to the directions on the package. Drain, then add the pasta to the tomato sauce and mix well using a pasta claw, or place individual servings of pasta in individual bowls and top with a lavish amount of tomato sauce. Garnish with nutritional yeast, if desired, and serve.

SERVES 4 TO 6

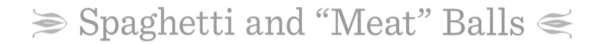

Spaghetti and "Meat" Balls

Don't be put off by the long ingredient list. Believe me, these
"meat" balls are well worth your effort!

¼ cup raw oatmeal

¼ cup cornmeal

⅛ cup whole-wheat or brown rice flour

1 teaspoon nutritional yeast flakes

¼ cup sunflower seeds

1 tablespoon dried oregano

1 tablespoon dried basil

1 teaspoon onion powder

1 teaspoon dry mustard

1 teaspoon chili powder

1 teaspoon paprika

1 teaspoon garlic powder

½ teaspoon salt

½ teaspoon freshly ground black
    pepper

⅛ teaspoon freshly grated nutmeg

½ cup canned adzuki beans or cooked
    green lentils

½ cup cooked brown rice

2 tablespoons olive oil

1 tablespoon powdered vegetable stock
    or equivalent in bouillon cubes,
    dissolved in ¼ cup boiling water

1 tablespoon soy sauce, tamari, or
    Braggs Liquid Aminos

1 tablespoon molasses

2 teaspoons lemon juice

1 teaspoon balsamic vinegar

1 teaspoon vegan Worcestershire
    sauce

6 button mushrooms, sliced very thin

1 pound spaghetti

1 recipe Tomato Sauce (from Pasta with
    Tomato Sauce, page 103)

Nutritional yeast flakes or commercially
    prepared vegan Parmesan cheese,
    for serving (optional)

Preheat the oven to 400°F. Grease a rimmed baking sheet.

Place the oatmeal, cornmeal, flour, nutritional yeast, sunflower seeds, oregano, basil, onion powder, dry mustard, chili powder, paprika, garlic powder, salt, pepper, and nutmeg in a large bowl. Mix well, then pour the mixture into the bowl of a food processor. Add the beans, rice, olive oil, stock, soy sauce, molasses, lemon juice, vinegar, and Worcestershire sauce and process, taking care not to overprocess; the texture of the mixture should be chunky. Add the mushrooms and pulse a few times.

Transfer the mixture to a large bowl. Using your hands, form the mixture into small balls, approximately 1 inch in diameter (larger balls will not cook through), and place them on the prepared baking sheet. Bake for 15 to 20 minutes, until golden brown. Remove from the oven and set aside. The "meat" balls are best when they have dried out somewhat (not fresh from the oven).

Prepare the pasta according to the directions on the package. Drain, then mix with the tomato sauce and top with the "meat" balls. Garnish with nutritional yeast, if desired.

SERVES 4 TO 6

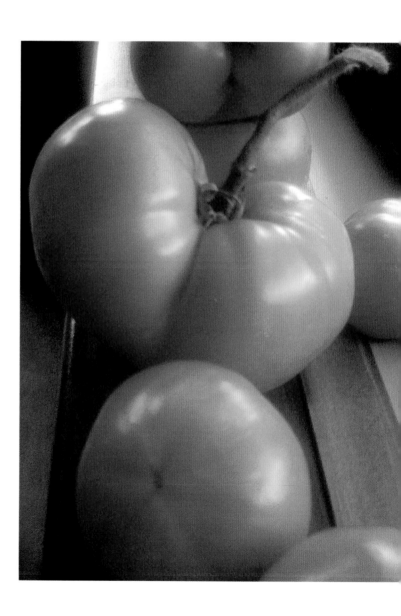

⋙ Creamy Mushroom Pasta ⋘

This pasta dish is deep and rich like the wild forest.

½ cup olive oil

10 ounces fresh mushrooms, any kind,
sliced thin

3 cloves garlic, finely chopped

1 tablespoon concentrated mushroom
broth or equivalent in bouillon cubes,
dissolved in ¼ cup boiling water

1 teaspoon truffle oil

½ cup water

2 tablespoons pastry flour (or use a
gluten-free alternative, like rice flour
or chestnut flour)

½ cup soy milk, rice milk, almond milk,
or coconut milk

Salt and coarsely ground black
pepper to taste

1 pound pasta, any kind

In a large frying pan, heat the olive oil over medium-high heat. Add the mushrooms and garlic and sauté, stirring often, for 5 to 6 minutes, until the mushrooms are soft. Reduce the heat to low and add the broth, truffle oil, and water. Stirring continuously, alternate adding small amounts of pastry flour and soy milk to create a gravy-like consistency. Reduce the heat to low and cook for 3 to 5 minutes. Using an immersion blender, blend until creamy. Add salt and pepper to taste.

Prepare the pasta according to the directions on the package. Drain, then mix with the sauce.

SERVES 4 TO 6

Mushroom and White Bean Pasta, Tuscan Style

The first time I had a dish like this was in a restaurant in a family home outside of Florence. The chef prepared one meal per day, and diners ate whatever meal was served—no menus! This recipe is my attempt to re-create that amazing repast. Note: *Farfalle* is an Italian word meaning "butterfly." It is often referred to as bow-tie pasta. Because of its shape, this pasta is especially good with a creamy sauce like this one.

½ cup olive oil

4 medium to large cloves garlic, finely chopped

4 teaspoons finely chopped fresh rosemary

6 large portabella mushrooms, sliced thin

One 16-ounce can cannellini beans, with their liquid

Salt and freshly ground black pepper to taste

½ cup water

¼ cup finely chopped fresh parsley

1 pound farfalle

In a large frying pan, heat the olive oil over medium-high heat. Add the garlic and rosemary and sauté for 3 minutes, stirring often. Add the mushrooms, reduce the heat to medium, and cook for 8 to 10 minutes. Add the beans with their liquid and salt and pepper to taste and stir to combine. Add the water, cover the pan, and simmer for another 5 minutes. Remove from the heat and mix in the parsley.

Prepare the pasta according to the directions on the package, drain, and mix with the sauce.

SERVES 4 TO 6

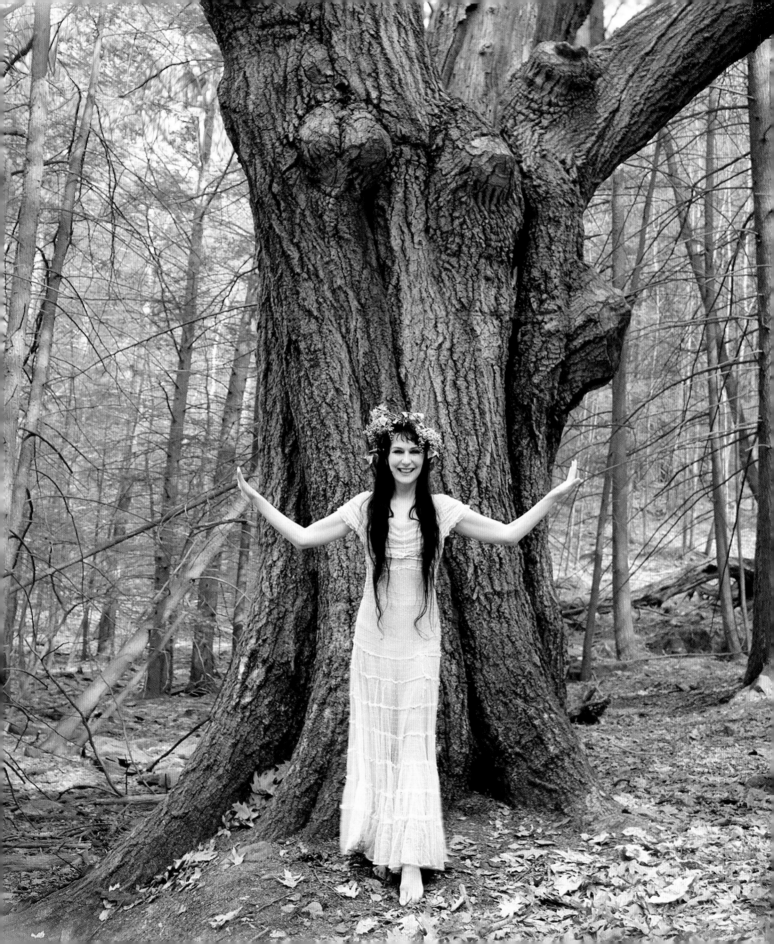

⇝ Wild Chanterelle Pasta ⇜

I developed this recipe when I discovered these small, golden, trumpet-shaped
mushrooms growing wild at the base of the oak trees in the forest where I live.
This sauce is also good over rice or kasha.

1 pound fresh chanterelle mushrooms,
   sliced thin, or 3 ounces dried
   chanterelle mushrooms

¼ cup olive oil

4 cloves garlic, chopped

½ onion, diced

2 teaspoons dried rosemary

1 tablespoon nutritional yeast flakes

¼ cup soy milk or almond milk

Salt and freshly ground black pepper
   to taste

1 pound pasta, any kind

If using dried mushrooms, place them in a small bowl, add boiling water to cover, and let stand
for about 20 minutes to rehydrate. Drain, reserving the soaking liquid, and slice the mushrooms.

In a large frying pan, heat the olive oil over medium heat. Add the garlic, onion, and rosemary
and sauté for 5 to 10 minutes, until the onions are translucent. Add the mushrooms and sauté
for another 5 minutes. In a cup, stir the nutritional yeast into the soy milk to dissolve, add the reserved soaking water if the mushrooms were rehydrated, then add the mixture to the frying pan.
Reduce the heat to low and simmer, covered, for 5 minutes. Add salt and pepper to taste.

Prepare the pasta according to the directions on the package. Drain, then mix with the sauce.

SERVES 4 TO 6

⪼ Faux Chicken Pasta ⪻

Chicken of the woods is a wild mushroom with a texture and taste very similar to chicken (as in the bird). This mushroom can be hard to find unless you have access to a forest of oak trees, so feel free to substitute commercially prepared faux chicken patties or strips, or any kind of mushroom, wild or tame, to make this delicious sautéed pasta dish.

⅓ cup olive oil, plus more as
needed
1 large yellow onion, sliced into thin
rounds
2 tablespoons dried tarragon

10 ounces chicken of the woods
mushrooms, sliced thin
1 pound pasta, any kind
Salt to taste
Red pepper flakes to taste

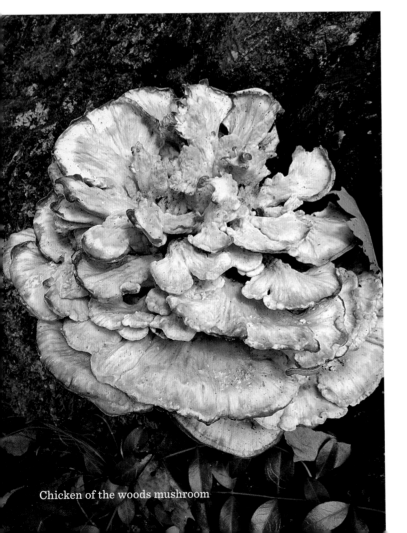

Chicken of the woods mushroom

In a large frying pan, heat the olive oil over medium-high heat. Add the onions and tarragon and sauté for 5 to 10 minutes, until the onions are translucent. Remove the onions and tarragon with a slotted spoon and set aside, leaving the oil in the pan. Add the mushrooms to the hot oil (adding more oil if necessary), sauté for a few minutes, then add back the onions and tarragon. Reduce the heat to medium and cook, stirring occasionally, until well mixed and heated throughout.

Prepare the pasta according to the directions on the package. Drain and mix in the sautéed mixture. Sprinkle with salt and red pepper flakes to taste.

SERVES 6 TO 8

⇒ Very Simple Glass Noodles ⇐

The taste of this dish is more complex than the simplicity of the recipe would suggest.

6 cups water

1 bunch spinach, kale, or collard greens
    (5 to 6 cups loosely packed)

2 ounces saifun noodles

1 tablespoon toasted sesame oil

1 tablespoon soy sauce, tamari,
    or Braggs Liquid Aminos

Red pepper flakes to taste

In a large pot, bring the water to a boil over high heat.

While the water is heating, wash the greens and chop them into small pieces. Place the greens in a stainless-steel pasta strainer or simple wire strainer.

Add the noodles to the boiling water and boil for about 2 minutes, until soft and clear then drain through the strainer over the greens. The hot water will "cook" the greens.

After straining, transfer the noodles and greens back into the empty pot. Using a pair of kitchen scissors, cut the noodles into smaller pieces. Pour the sesame oil and soy sauce over the noodles and greens and mix well using a pasta claw. Sprinkle with red pepper flakes to taste.

SERVES 2

⇒ Dressed-Up Glass Noodles ⇐

This recipe contains a mélange of contrasts—sweet and savory,
soft and crunchy, green and yellow, red and white.

6 to 8 sun-dried tomatoes

6 cups water

2 tablespoons toasted sesame oil, plus
more to taste

Two 6-inch-long commercially prepared
vegan sausages, cut into small discs

½ apple, cored and chopped into small
pieces

1 bunch spinach, kale, or collard greens,
chopped into small pieces (5 to
6 cups loosely packed)

½ cup fresh, frozen, or canned corn
kernels

2 ounces saifun noodles

Soy sauce, tamari, or Braggs Liquid
Aminos to taste

In a small bowl, place the tomatoes, add boiling water to cover, and let stand for about 10 minutes, until the tomatoes are rehydrated. Drain the tomatoes and discard the soaking liquid. Using kitchen scissors, cut the rehydrated tomatoes into thin strips and set aside.

In a large pot, bring the water to a boil over high heat. While the water is heating, in a medium frying pan, heat the sesame oil over medium-high heat. Add the sausages and sauté for about 3 minutes, turning once, until well heated and starting to brown. Add the tomatoes and apple and cook for 1 more minute, then remove from the heat.

Place the greens and corn in a stainless-steel pasta strainer or simple wire strainer. Add the noodles to the boiling water and boil for about 2 minutes, until soft and clear, then drain them through the strainer over the greens and corn. The hot water will "cook" the greens and corn.

After straining, transfer the noodles, greens, and corn back into the empty pot. Using kitchen scissors, cut the noodles into smaller pieces. Add the sautéed mixture to the pot and mix well. Add more sesame oil and soy sauce to taste.

SERVES 2 TO 4

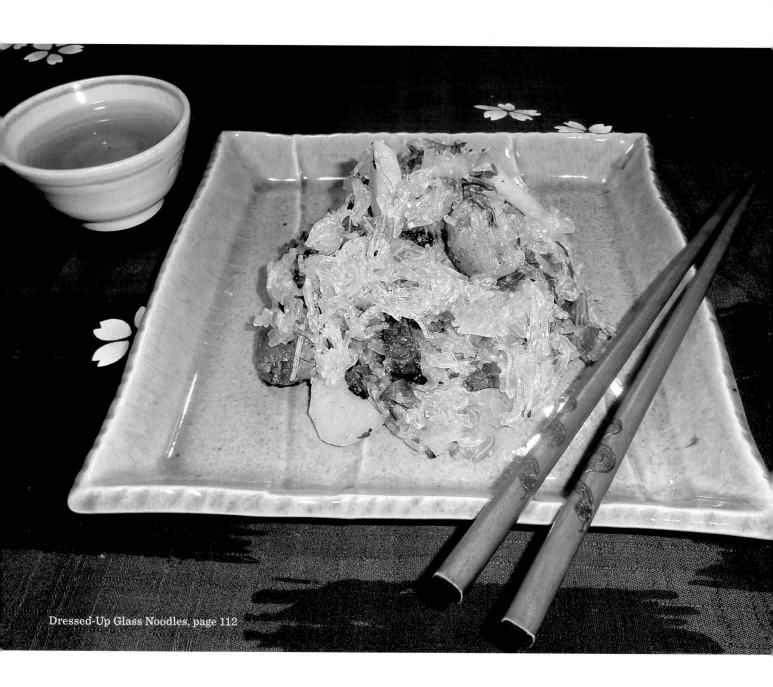

Dressed-Up Glass Noodles, page 112

⪢ Deluxe Asian Noodles ⪡

This is a versatile stir-fry. Feel free to substitute any vegetables that you have on hand.

4 dried shiitake mushrooms

¼ cup dried hijiki seaweed

2 tablespoons rice vinegar

3 tablespoons toasted sesame oil, plus
   more to taste

1 tablespoon soy sauce, tamari, or
   Braggs Liquid Aminos, plus more to
   taste

1 teaspoon agave

6 to 8 cups water, depending on the
   amount of noodles used

12 to 16 ounces soba, udon, rice
   noodles, or saifun noodles

One ½-inch piece fresh ginger, peeled
   and finely chopped

1 clove garlic, finely chopped

½ teaspoon red pepper flakes

3 ounces commercially prepared baked
   tofu, cut into small cubes

1 carrot, peeled and cut into small
   pieces

3 leaves and stalks bok choy, finely
   chopped

3 stalks celery, chopped into diagonal
   slices

6 ounces mung bean sprouts

1 cup firmly packed fresh spinach

In a large bowl, place the mushrooms and seaweed, add boiling water to cover, and let stand for 5 to 10 minutes, until the mushrooms are soft. Drain the mushrooms and seaweed, reserving the soaking liquid. Remove the mushrooms from the bowl, slice them into thin strips, and set aside.

To the bowl that contains the rehydrated seaweed, add the vinegar, 1 tablespoon of the sesame oil, the soy sauce, and the agave. Allow the seaweed to marinate for at least 10 minutes or up to 1 hour.

In a large soup pot, bring the water to a boil over high heat. Add the noodles and cook according to the package directions. Drain well and set aside.

In a large frying pan or wok, heat the remaining 2 tablespoons sesame oil. Add the ginger, garlic, and red pepper flakes and sauté for 2 to 3 minutes, until fragrant. Add the mushrooms, tofu, carrot, bok choy, and celery and stir-fry for about 3 minutes, until well heated and starting to get soft. Add the noodles, marinated seaweed, reserved soaking liquid, sprouts, and spinach to the frying pan and mix well. Drizzle sesame oil and soy sauce over the noodles to taste.

SERVES 4 TO 6

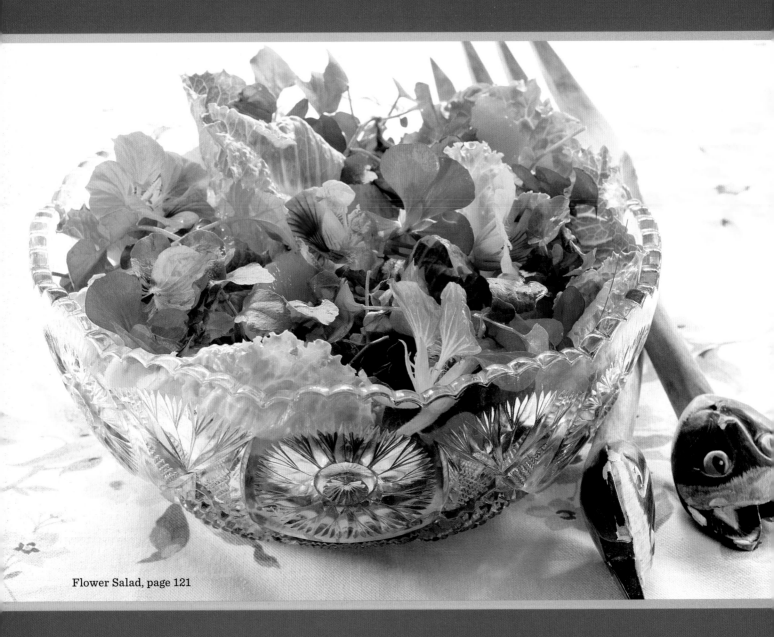

Flower Salad, page 121

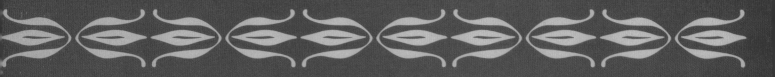

Salads

A mixture of predominately raw vegetables arranged in an aesthetically pleasing way, a salad can be eaten alone as a main course or as a starter or side dish. Salads are usually mixed with a dressing, but some purists prefer their salads "dry." They say they can taste the vegetables better without getting distracted. Salads are usually served for lunch or dinner, but they can be eaten for breakfast by the adventuresome.

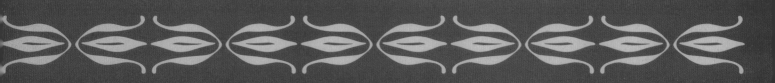

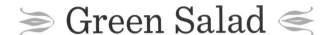 Green Salad

10 leaves red-leaf lettuce, green-leaf
    lettuce, iceberg lettuce, or romaine
    lettuce, chopped or torn into pieces
1 handful mesclun salad mix, or 2 to
    3 leaves curly endive, chopped or
    torn into pieces
5 leaves fresh basil, chopped or torn
    into pieces

1 tomato, chopped
Dressing of your choice (see
    pages 152–160)
Salt and freshly ground black pepper
    to taste

Place lettuce, mesclun, basil, and tomato in a bowl and mix well. Toss with dressing and salt and pepper to taste.

SERVES 1 TO 4

Endive and Walnut Salad

1 bunch curly endive, chopped
   (8 to 12 cups loosely packed)
1 tomato, chopped, or 6 cherry
   tomatoes
2 tablespoons olive oil
8 walnuts, halved

1 teaspoon agave
The Most Simple Dressing (page 152)
   or any other dressing (see
   pages 152–160) to taste
Salt and freshly ground black pepper
   to taste

Place the endive and tomato in a large bowl.

In a small frying pan, heat the olive oil over medium heat. Add the walnuts and sauté for 3 minutes, stirring continuously, taking care not to let the walnuts burn. Pour the agave over the walnuts and stir for a few seconds. Remove from the pan and place on a brown paper bag to drain for a few minutes, until dry. Add the walnuts, dressing, and salt and pepper to taste and toss.

SERVES 1 TO 4

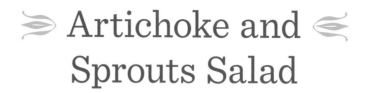 Artichoke and Sprouts Salad

1 romaine heart, or ½ head iceberg
    lettuce, cut in a thin chiffonade
One 10-ounce can or jar artichokes,
    liquid drained, chopped into quarters
½ cup fresh or canned corn
1 cup alfalfa, clover, or mixed sprouts

The Most Simple Dressing (page 152)
    or any other dressing (see
    pages 152–160) to taste
Salt and freshly ground black pepper
    to taste

In a large bowl, place the lettuce, artichokes, corn, and sprouts and mix well. Toss with the dressing and salt and pepper to taste.

SERVES 1 TO 4

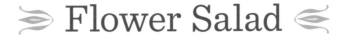 Flower Salad

This is definitely a seasonal salad. Nasturtium and bergamot bloom only in late summer.

1 large handful mixed salad greens

1 orange, peeled and separated into sections

½ cucumber, peeled and sliced thin

5 to 10 bergamot flowers

5 to 10 nasturtium flowers

¼ cup commercially prepared vegan Cheddar cheese, shredded

Dressing of your choice (see pages 152–160) to taste

Arrange the greens, orange, cucumber, flowers, and cheese harmoniously in a large bowl and top with dressing to taste.

SERVES 1 TO 4

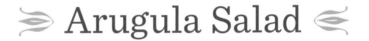 Arugula Salad

1 bunch arugula, chopped

¼ cup commercially prepared vegan Cheddar cheese, shredded

3 green or black pitted olives, thinly sliced

The Most Simple Dressing (page 152) or any other dressing (see pages 152–160) to taste

Salt and freshly ground black pepper to taste

¼ avocado, thinly sliced

Combine the arugula, cheese, and olives in a large bowl. Toss with the dressing and salt and pepper to taste, then harmoniously arrange the sliced avocados on top.

SERVES 1 TO 4

⇒ Arugula and Mustard Salad ⇐

1 bunch arugula, chopped

6 large leaves mustard greens, chopped

2 leaves romaine lettuce or green-leaf
lettuce, chopped

2 slices red onion, finely chopped

3 cherry tomatoes, cut into quarters

Dressing of your choice (see
pages 152–160) to taste

Salt and freshly ground black pepper
to taste

Combine the arugula, mustard greens, romaine, onion, and tomatoes in a large bowl. Toss with
the dressing and salt and pepper to taste.

SERVES 1 TO 4

⇒ Green Leaves and ⇐ Sweet Pepper Salad

½ romaine heart and an equal amount
arugula, chopped

½ red or yellow bell pepper, cut into
small pieces

The Most Simple Dressing (page 152) or
any other dressing (see
pages 152–160) to taste

Salt and freshly ground black pepper
to taste

In a large bowl, combine the greens and bell pepper. Toss with the dressing and salt and pepper to
taste.

SERVES 1 TO 4

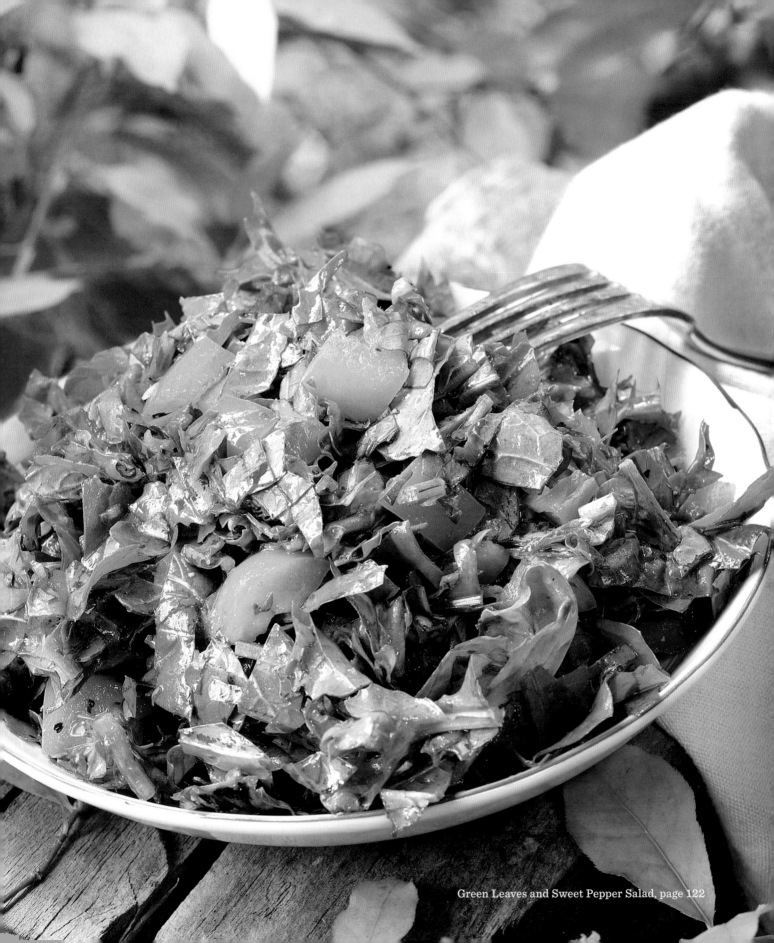

Green Leaves and Sweet Pepper Salad, page 122

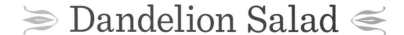 Dandelion Salad

1 bunch fresh dandelion greens,
  chopped
4 leaves red-leaf lettuce, chopped
1 tomato, chopped

Dressing of your choice (see
  pages 152–160) to taste
Salt and freshly ground black pepper
  to taste

Combine the dandelion greens, lettuce, and tomato in a large bowl. Toss with the dressing and salt and pepper to taste.

SERVES 1 TO 4

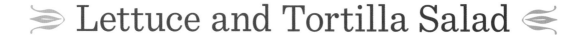 Lettuce and Tortilla Salad

½ head iceberg lettuce, chopped
1 large tomato, cut into small
  pieces
¼ sweet red onion, finely chopped
2 handfuls corn tortilla chips

Mustard Dressing (page 159) or any
  other dressing (see pages 152–160)
  to taste
Salt and freshly ground black pepper
  to taste

Combine the lettuce, tomato, onion, and corn chips in a large bowl. Toss with the dressing and salt and pepper to taste.

SERVES 1 TO 4

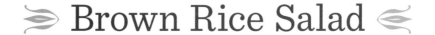 Brown Rice Salad

This is a meal in itself.

2 cups cooked brown rice

One 8-ounce package firm tofu,
   cut into cubes

½ onion, finely chopped

6 large leaves red-leaf lettuce or
   romaine lettuce, torn or cut into
   small pieces

2 sheets nori, cut into thin strips with
   scissors

Turmeric-Tahini Dressing (page 159)
   or any other dressing (see pages
   152–160) to taste

Salt and freshly ground black pepper
   to taste

Combine the rice, tofu, onion, lettuce, and nori in a large bowl. Toss with the dressing and salt
and pepper to taste.

SERVES 1 TO 4

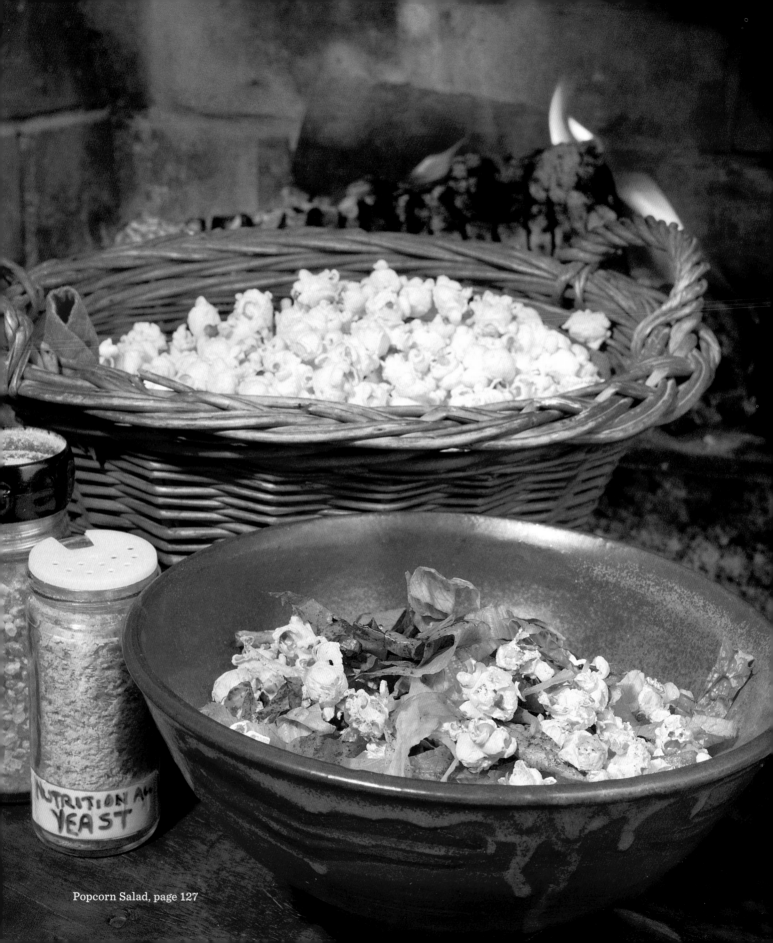

Popcorn Salad, page 127

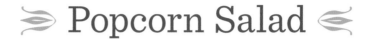 Popcorn Salad

What could be more fun than making a salad with popcorn as the main ingredient?

1 cup popped popcorn

1 tablespoon nutritional yeast flakes

1 teaspoon flaxseed oil

¼ teaspoon red pepper flakes

½ teaspoon salt

½ head iceberg lettuce, or 1 romaine
   heart, finely chopped

1 tomato, cut into small pieces

1 scallion, finely chopped

Dressing of your choice (see
   pages 152–160) to taste

In a large bowl, place the popcorn, nutritional yeast, flaxseed oil, red pepper flakes, and salt and mix well to coat evenly. Add the lettuce, tomato, and scallion and mix well. Toss with the dressing.

SERVES 1 TO 4

❧ Caesar Salad ❧

Once you try this Caesar, you'll never go back to cheese, eggs, and anchovies.

1 romaine heart, torn or cut into small pieces

¼ cup Tempeh Croutons (page 200)

6 pitted kalamata olives, cut into small pieces

1 tablespoon hulled sunflower seeds

1 tablespoon nutritional yeast flakes

Caesar Dressing (page 157) to taste

Salt and freshly ground black pepper to taste

Combine the lettuce, croutons, olives, sunflower seeds, and nutritional yeast in a large bowl. Toss with the dressing and salt and pepper to taste.

SERVES 1 TO 4

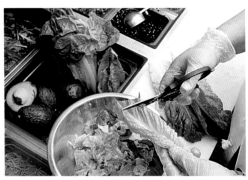

1.

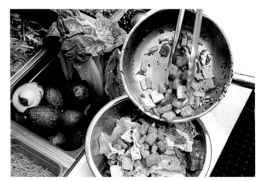

2.

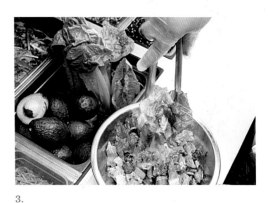

3.

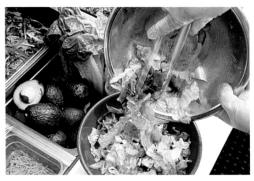

4.

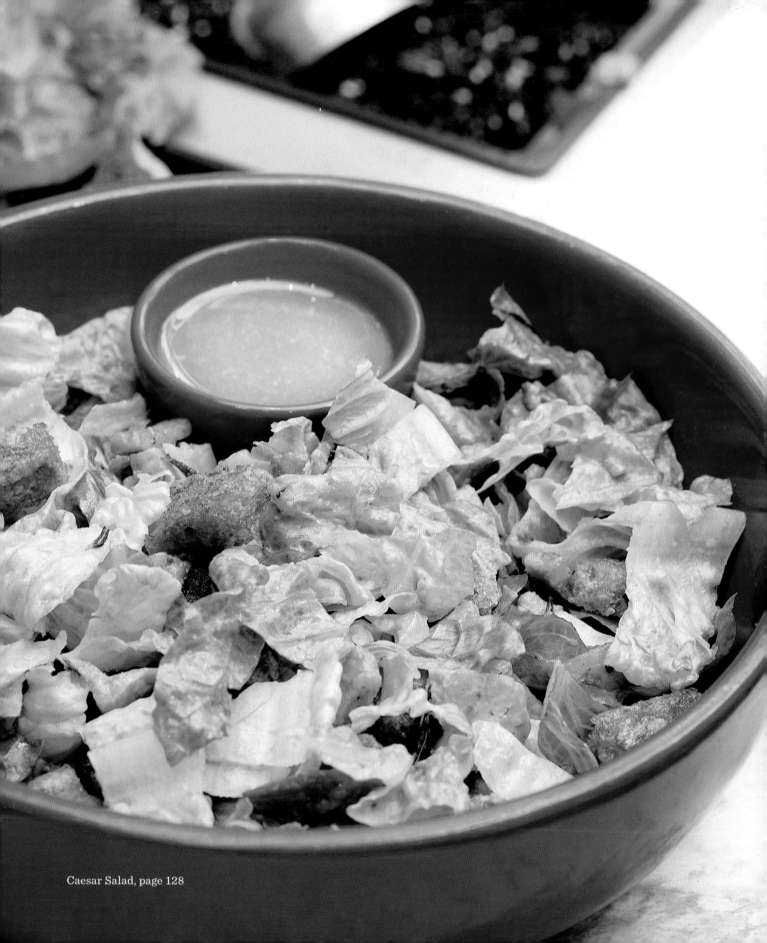

Caesar Salad, page 128

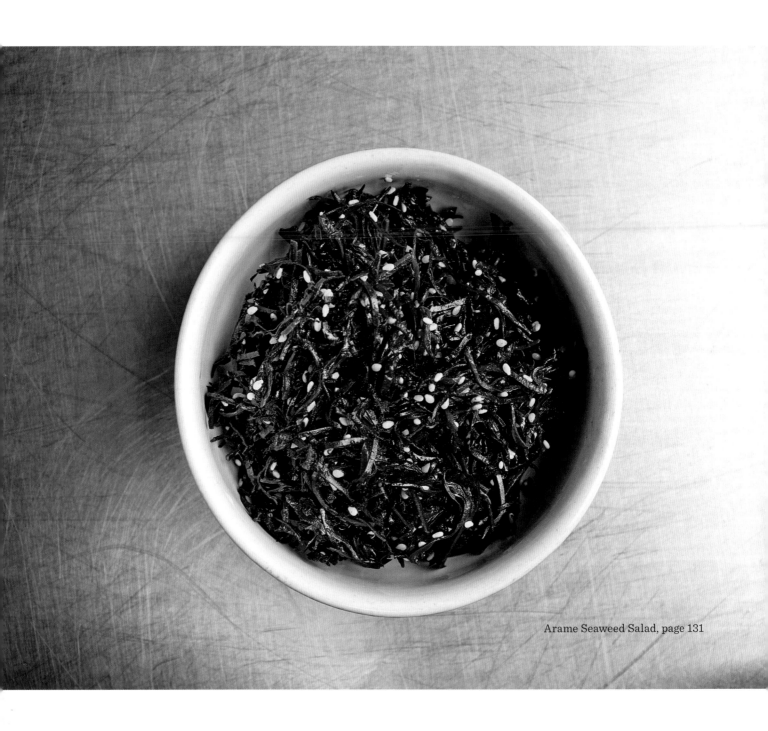

Arame Seaweed Salad, page 131

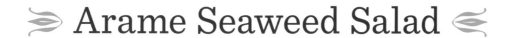 Arame Seaweed Salad

A favorite at Jivamuktea Café. Arame is high in minerals, especially calcium.
If you're not familiar with seaweed, you're in for a real treat!

¼ cup dried arame seaweed

½ cup water

½ tablespoon toasted sesame oil

1 teaspoon soy sauce, tamari, or Braggs Liquid Aminos

1 teaspoon sesame seeds

In a small saucepan, place the seaweed and water, cover, and bring to a boil over high heat. Reduce the heat to low and simmer for 10 to 15 minutes, until the seaweed is tender. Drain, then transfer the seaweed to a bowl. Add the sesame oil, soy sauce, and sesame seeds and mix well. Enjoy immediately or store in a tightly sealed container for up to 1 week in the refrigerator.

SERVES 1 TO 4

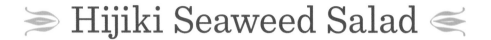 Hijiki Seaweed Salad

This salad is a sweet-and-sour delight.

¼ cup dried hijiki seaweed

½ cup boiling water

1 teaspoon toasted sesame oil

1 teaspoon mirin

1 teaspoon brown rice vinegar

1 teaspoon agave

1 teaspoon soy sauce, tamari, or Braggs
Liquid Aminos

In a small bowl, place the seaweed, add the boiling water to cover and let stand for 5 to 10 minutes to rehydrate. Add the sesame oil, mirin, vinegar, agave, and soy sauce and stir well. Enjoy immediately or store in a tightly sealed container for up to 1 week in the refrigerator.

SERVES 1 TO 4

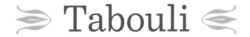

Tabouli

Despite ingredients like wheat and nuts, this concoction is surprisingly light and fresh.

2¼ cups water

1 cup bulgur wheat

¼ cup chopped walnuts

2 tomatoes, finely chopped

2 scallions (white and green parts only), sliced thin

3¼ cups fresh cilantro, chopped

2 cloves garlic, finely chopped

Juice of 1 lemon

2 tablespoons olive oil

1 teaspoon ground cumin

Salt and freshly ground black pepper to taste

In a medium saucepan, bring the water to a boil. Stir in the bulgur, cover, turn off the heat, and let the bulgur sit for 30 minutes to absorb the water. Drain any liquid left unabsorbed.

In a large salad bowl, place the bulgur, walnuts, tomatoes, scallions, cilantro, garlic, lemon juice, olive oil, and cumin and mix well. Season with salt and pepper to taste. Refrigerate for at least 3 hours to blend the flavors. Serve cold.

FOR ALTERNATIVE FLAVORS, TRY

- pine nuts instead of walnuts
- parsley instead of cilantro
- quinoa instead of bulgur wheat
- 1 cup prepared Spirulina Millet (page 180) instead of cooked bulgur wheat
- ½ red onion, finely chopped, instead of scallions, or leave the onions out altogether

SERVES 1 TO 4

❧ Very Simple ❧
Shredded Beet Salad

1 large raw beet, peeled and shredded

1 tablespoon lemon juice

Salt to taste

In a bowl, place the shredded beet and mix in the lemon juice and salt to taste. Chill for at least 30 minutes before serving.

SERVES 1 TO 4

❧ Shredded Beet ❧
and Carrot Salad

1 large raw beet, peeled and shredded

1 large carrot, peeled and shredded

4 walnuts, chopped

2 tablespoons raisins

1 teaspoon balsamic vinegar

2 tablespoons olive oil

Salt and freshly ground black pepper
   to taste

In a bowl, place the shredded beet and carrot. Add the walnuts, raisins, vinegar, olive oil, and salt and pepper to taste. Mix lightly so as to retain the separate red and orange colors. Chill for at least 30 minutes before serving.

SERVES 1 TO 4

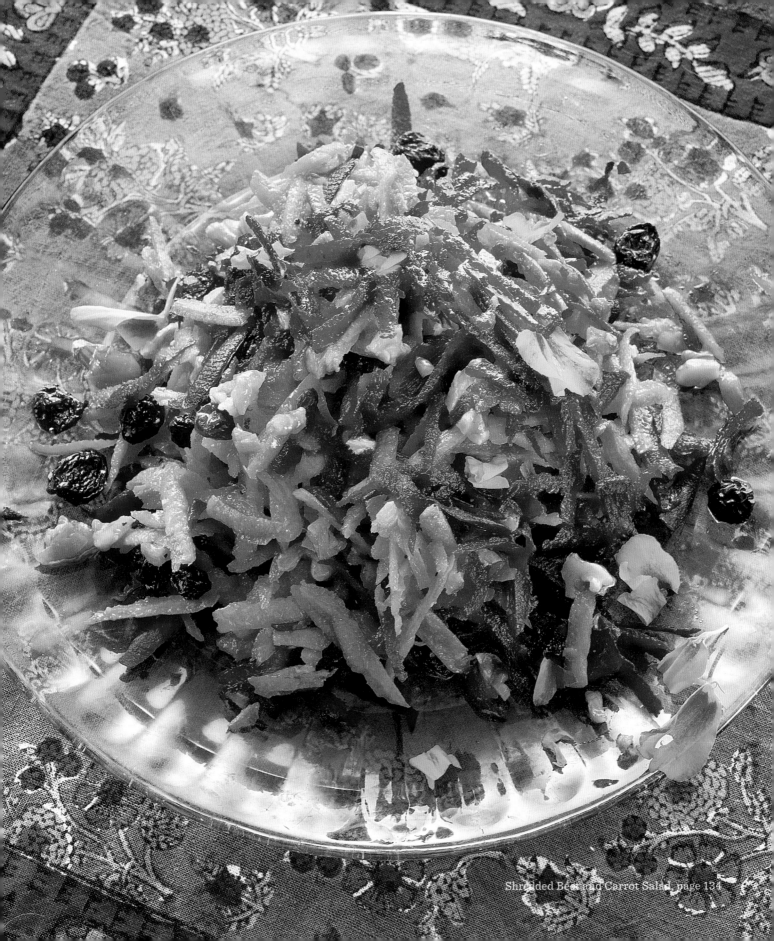

Shredded Beet and Carrot Salad, page 134

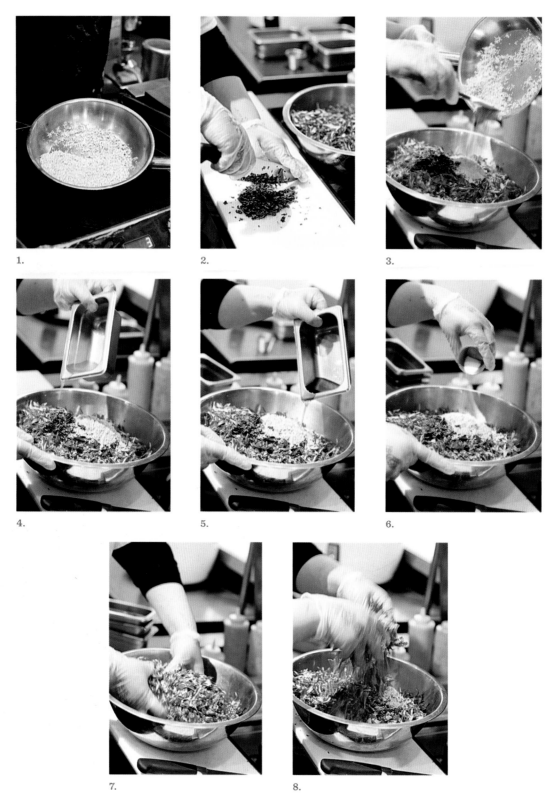

1.

2.

3.

4.

5.

6.

7.

8.

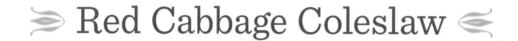

Red Cabbage Coleslaw

The "cole" in "coleslaw" comes from the Dutch word for cabbage. To keep up with demand for this popular salad at Jivamuktea Café, our chefs have to triple or quadruple the recipe.

1 tablespoon sesame seeds
½ head red cabbage, stemmed and cut
   in a thin chiffonade
¼ bunch fresh cilantro, stems removed
   and leaves finely chopped

¼ cup brown rice vinegar
3 tablespoons toasted sesame oil
1 tablespoon agave
½ teaspoon salt

Heat a small frying pan over medium heat. Add the sesame seeds to the hot pan and toast for 3 minutes.

In a large mixing bowl, place the cabbage, cilantro, vinegar, sesame oil, agave, salt, and toasted sesame seeds and mix well. Adjust the seasonings so that the coleslaw is not too sweet and all the flavors come through. The coleslaw should be slightly more vinegary than oily.

SERVES 1 TO 4

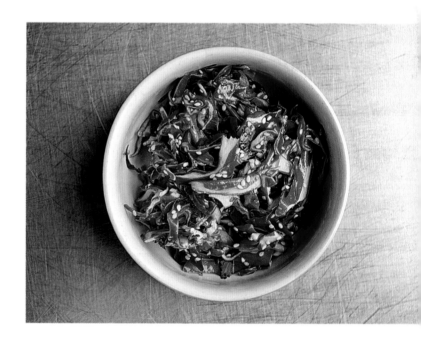

Fat-Free Super-Simple Snow Cone Cabbage Salad

This salad, as light as snow, will make you forget you're dieting!

2 cups coarsely chopped white cabbage

2 tablespoons lemon juice

½ cucumber, chopped into small pieces

½ teaspoon salt

Paprika to taste

In the bowl of a food processor, place the cabbage, lemon juice, cucumber, and salt and process until the cabbage is very finely shredded, resembling a snow cone. Using a rubber spatula, remove the salad and place it in small individual serving bowls. Sprinkle with paprika to taste.

SERVES 1 TO 4

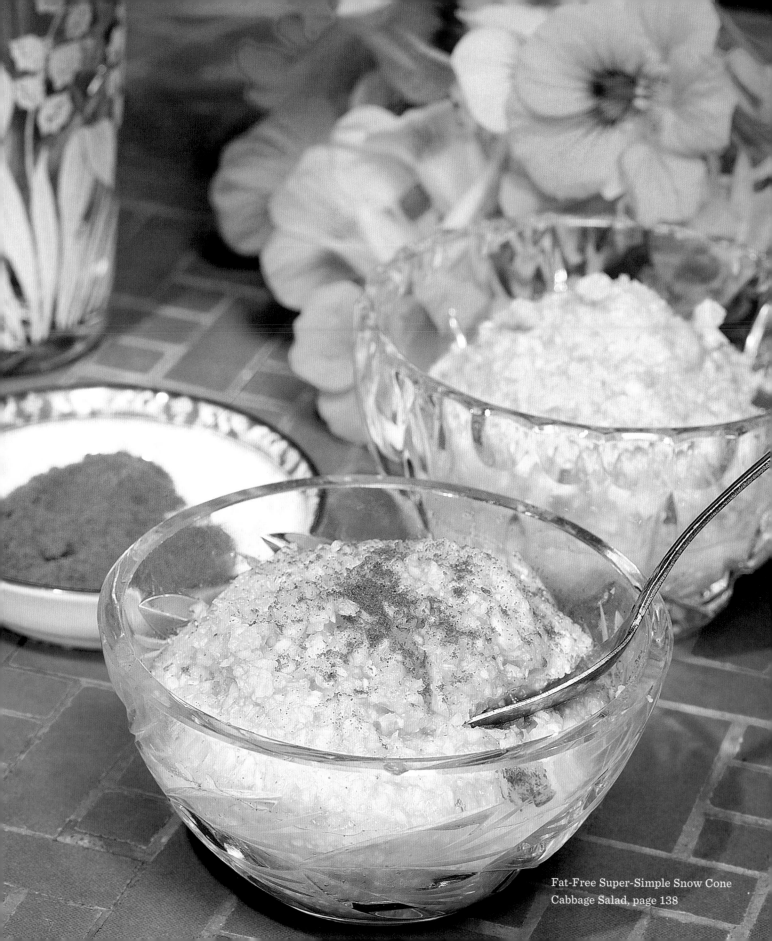

Fat-Free Super-Simple Snow Cone
Cabbage Salad, page 138

Black Sesame Seed Cabbage Slaw

The color, in addition to the flavor of the toasted sesame oil,

makes this salad especially appetizing.

2 cups coarsely chopped white cabbage

2 tablespoons toasted sesame oil

2 tablespoons lemon juice

1 tablespoon vegan mayonnaise

1 teaspoon stone-ground mustard

1 teaspoon ground cumin

½ teaspoon salt

1 cup raw mung bean sprouts, coarsely
   chopped

¼ cup finely chopped fresh parsley

2 tablespoons black sesame seeds

In the bowl of a food processor, place the cabbage, sesame oil, lemon juice, mayonnaise, mustard, cumin, and salt and process until the cabbage is finely chopped. Transfer to a large bowl and stir in the sprouts, parsley, and sesame seeds.

SERVES 1 TO 4

Potato-Zucchini Salad

Traditional potato salad is often too heavy for my taste, so I lighten
it with zucchini, green beans, and parsley.

4 medium to large potatoes, chopped
into ½-inch cubes

1 medium to large zucchini, chopped
into ½-inch cubes

12 French-style green beans, chopped
into ½-inch pieces

¼ cup very finely chopped fresh parsley

Vegan mayonnaise to taste

Lemon juice to taste

Salt and freshly ground black pepper
to taste

In a steamer basket set over boiling water, place the potatoes and zucchini and steam for about 20 minutes, until soft. Add the green beans and steam for another 3 to 5 minutes; the green beans should be crisp and still retain their color. Transfer the steamed vegetables to a large bowl and place in the refrigerator to chill for about 1 hour, until cold. Stir in the parsley. Add the mayonnaise, lemon juice, and salt and pepper to taste.

SERVES 4 TO 6

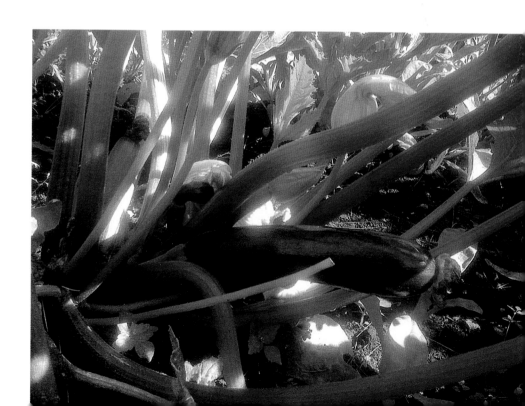

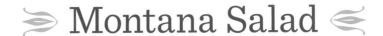 Montana Salad

This is the all-time best-selling menu item at Jivamuktea Café.

2½ cups mesclun salad mix

4 cherry tomatoes

¼ cup shredded carrots

½ cup cooked quinoa

½ cup cooked Black Beans (page 190)

¼ avocado, slice cut into ⅛-inch slices

Dressing of your choice (see
pages 152–160) to taste

In a large bowl, place the mesclun loosely and arrange the tomatoes at nine o'clock, the carrots at three o'clock, the quinoa at twelve o'clock, and the beans at six o'clock. Array the avocado slices in the center. Pour the dressing over the salad.

SERVES 1

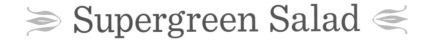 Supergreen Salad

The concentrated chlorophyll in the spirulina makes this salad "supergreen."

2½ cups mesclun salad mix

⅓ cup Red Cabbage Coleslaw
(page 137)

⅓ cup Spirulina Millet (page 180)

Dressing of your choice (see
pages 152–160) to taste

In a large bowl, place the mesclun loosely and layer the coleslaw on top of the greens, then nestle the millet in the center of the coleslaw. Pour the dressing over the salad.

SERVES 1

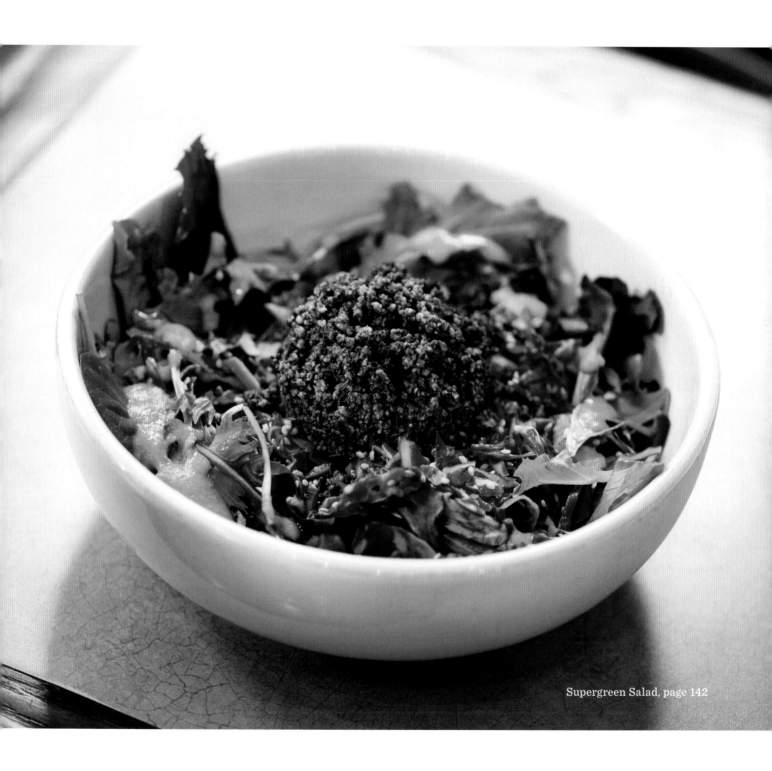

Supergreen Salad, page 142

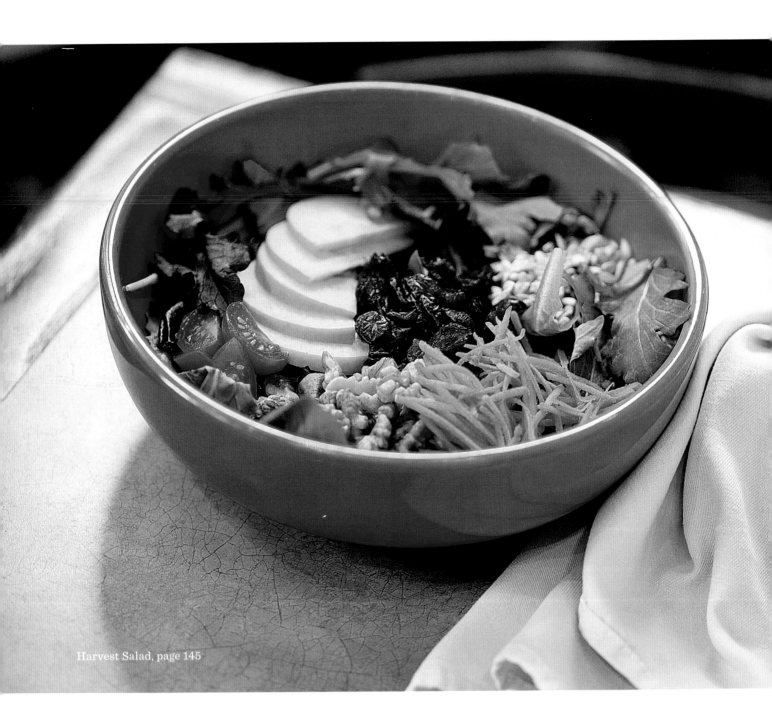
Harvest Salad, page 145

Harvest Salad
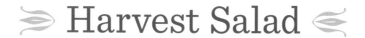

This gathering of fruit and nuts will energize you.

2½ cups mesclun salad mix

¼ cup shredded carrots

¼ cup chopped raw walnuts

1 tablespoon dried cranberries

2 tablespoons hulled sunflower seeds

4 cherry tomatoes

¼ Granny Smith apple, sliced thin

Dressing of your choice (see
    pages 152–160) to taste

In a large bowl, place the mesclun loosely and arrange the carrots at three o'clock, the walnuts at nine o'clock, the cranberries at six o'clock, and the sunflower seeds at twelve o'clock. Top each clock point with one tomato. Arrange the apple slices decoratively in the center. Pour the dressing over the salad.

SERVES 1

Spicy Tempeh Salad
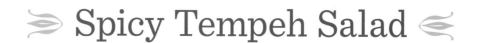

This protein-rich salad features tempeh generously seasoned with red pepper.

2½ cups mesclun salad mix

4 cherry tomatoes

¼ cup shredded carrots

4 ounces Tempeh Croutons (page 200)

Dressing of your choice (see
    pages 152–160) to taste

In a large bowl, place the mesclun loosely and arrange the tomatoes at nine o'clock, the carrots at three o'clock, and croutons in the center. Pour the dressing over the salad.

SERVES 1

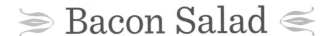 Bacon Salad

This salad is salty, rich, crunchy, sweet, and nourishing.

2½ cups mesclun salad mix

4 cherry tomatoes

¼ cup shredded carrots

3 strips commercially prepared tempeh
   bacon, grilled

6 kalamata olives

3 ounces Hummus (page 165)

Dressing of your choice (see
   pages 152–160) to taste

In a large bowl, place the mesclun loosely and arrange the tomatoes at nine o'clock, the carrots at three o'clock, the tempeh bacon at six o'clock, the olives at twelve o'clock, and the hummus in the center. Pour the dressing over the salad.

SERVES 1

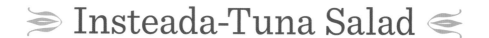

Insteada-Tuna Salad

Yes, normally tempeh is cooked, and this recipe calls for "uncooked" tempeh, but tempeh is actually not a raw food, though some may disagree. Here's the scoop: tempeh is made by fermenting already cooked soybeans with the mold *Rhizopus oligosporus*, but by the end of the fermentation there is not much left of the beans because the tempeh culture has "eaten" them and thus incorporated the nutrients and amino acids of the beans into its moldy body— mmmm, tasty! Enough said—this insteada-tuna salad is quick to make and is infinitely kinder to the fish, the oceans, the planet, and yourself.

12 ounces tempeh (uncooked)
½ cup vegan mayonnaise
½ cup brown rice vinegar
4 stalks celery, finely chopped
½ white onion, minced

½ teaspoon kelp powder
1 teaspoon dulse flakes
Salt and freshly ground black pepper
    to taste

In a large bowl, place the tempeh and mash it using your hands or a large fork. Add the mayonnaise, vinegar, celery, onion, kelp powder, dulse flakes, and salt and pepper to taste and mix well.

SERVES 2 TO 4

Marinated Tomato Salad

Use as a side dish to add zest and sweetness to any meal.

1 large tomato, cut into pieces, or
10 cherry tomatoes, halved
2 tablespoons balsamic vinegar

1 tablespoon agave
Dash of salt

In a small bowl, place the tomato, vinegar, agave, and salt and allow to sit for at least 20 minutes.

SERVES 1 TO 4

Marinated Beet Salad

The sweet-and-sour tang and deep red color are to die for!

4 beets, unpeeled
1 cup balsamic vinegar
½ cup fresh cilantro, finely chopped

2 teaspoons olive oil
1 teaspoon salt
1 teaspoon freshly ground black pepper

In a steamer basket set over boiling water, place the beets and steam for about 1 hour, or until they are soft. Allow the beets to cool for about 5 minutes, until they are cool enough to handle, then peel off the skin and dice the beets into ½-inch pieces. Place the diced beets in a medium bowl or large jar. Add the vinegar, cilantro, olive oil, salt, and pepper and mix well. Cover and refrigerate for at least 1 hour.

SERVES 6 TO 8

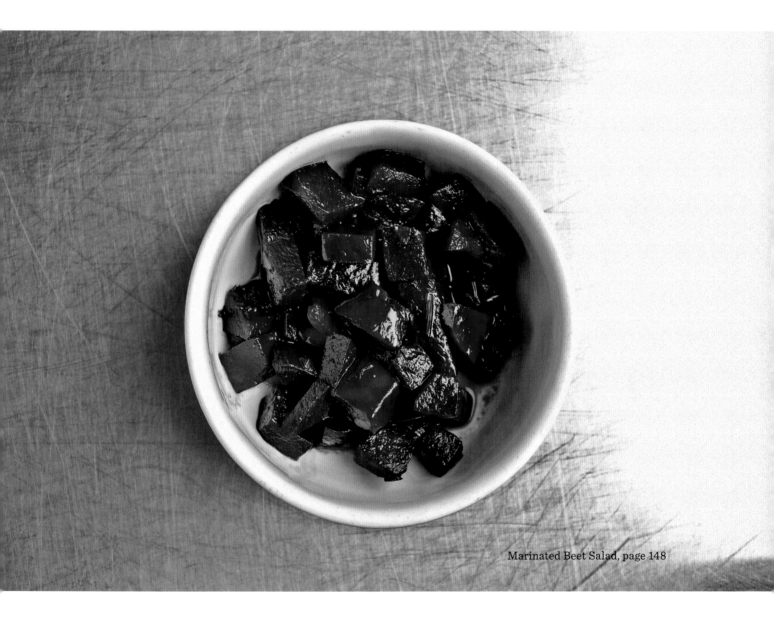

Marinated Beet Salad, page 148

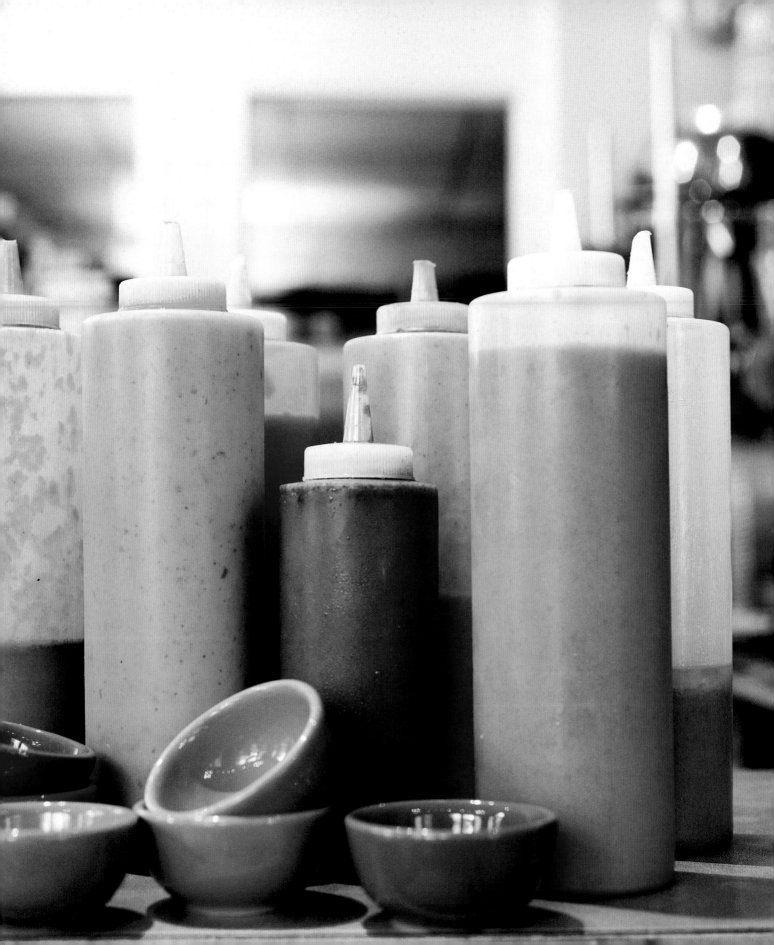

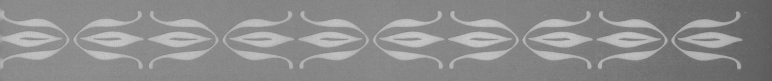

Dressings

These recipes are usually used to enhance the flavor of salads, but they can also serve as condiments for cooked or raw vegetables, beans, or grains.

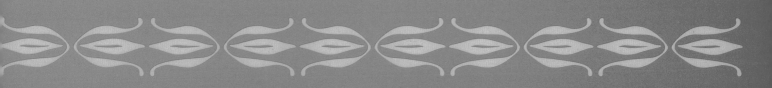

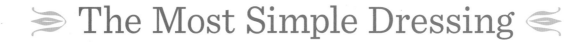

The Most Simple Dressing

Unlike most of the dressings in this chapter, this one is
not prepared separately from the salad it dresses.

2 tablespoons olive oil
1 tablespoon lemon juice
Salt and freshly ground black pepper to taste

Pour the olive oil over the salad first, and gently toss so that all leaves are coated. Add the lemon juice, sprinkle with salt and pepper to taste, then toss again.

MAKES 3 TABLESPOONS

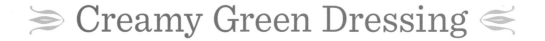

Creamy Green Dressing

½ cup olive oil

½ cup fresh parsley

1 tablespoon vegan mayonnaise

1 tablespoon lemon juice or lime juice

1 tablespoon prepared mustard

1 teaspoon spirulina powder

1 teaspoon agave

¾ cup water

In the bowl of a food processor or in a blender jar, place the olive oil, parsley, mayonnaise, lemon juice, mustard, spirulina, agave, and water and blend until smooth and very green.

MAKES 1½ CUPS

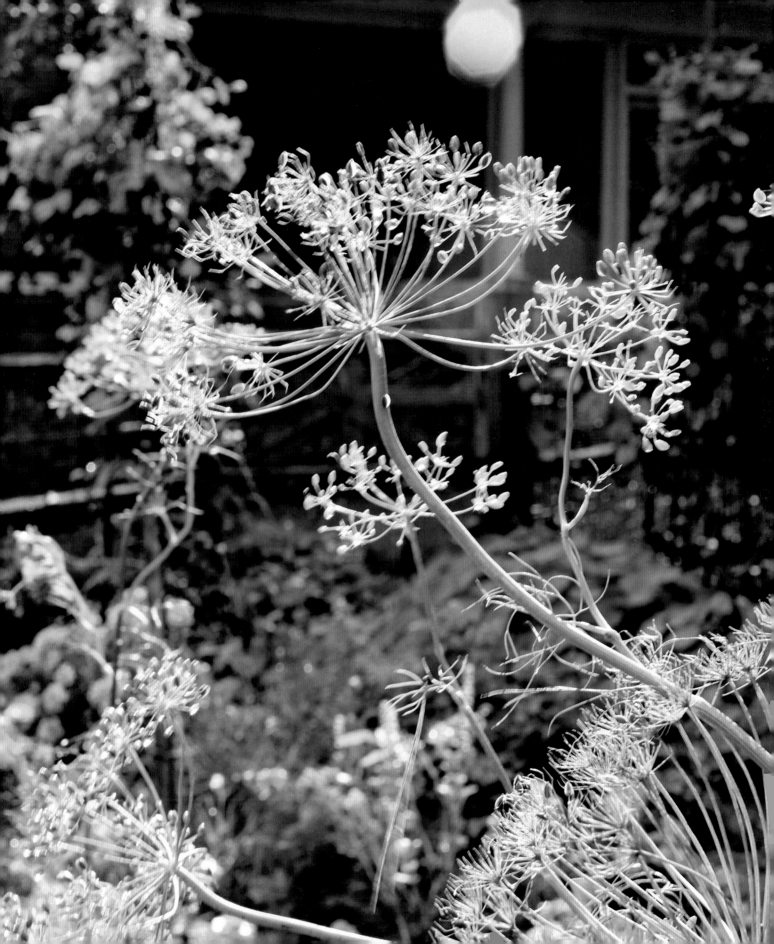

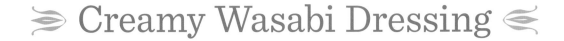 Creamy Wasabi Dressing

1 cup tahini

1 tablespoon wasabi powder

½ cup rice vinegar

½ cup soy sauce, tamari, or Braggs
Liquid Aminos

In the bowl of a food processor or in a blender jar, place the tahini, wasabi, vinegar, and soy sauce and blend until smooth.

MAKES 2 CUPS

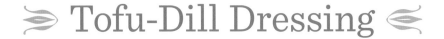 Tofu-Dill Dressing

½ cup cashews

Water, as needed

8 ounces soft tofu

2 tablespoons olive oil

1 tablespoon dried dill

1 tablespoon nutritional yeast flakes

1 tablespoon lemon juice

1 teaspoon agave

1 teaspoon brown rice vinegar

¼ teaspoon salt

In the bowl of a food processor, place the cashews and blend, adding a small amount of water if needed. Add the tofu, olive oil, dill, nutritional yeast, lemon juice, agave, vinegar, and salt and blend, adding more water as necessary to yield the consistency you want.

MAKES 1¼ CUPS

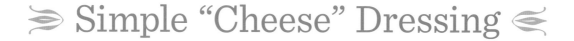 Simple "Cheese" Dressing

This sauce is great over broccoli, rice, kasha, or potatoes.

Just about anything tastes better with this sauce.

⅔ cup nutritional yeast flakes

¾ to 1 cup water

2 tablespoons olive oil

2 tablespoons chickpea miso or mellow white miso

2 tablespoons tahini, cashew butter, or almond butter

1 tablespoon dried sage or oregano

1 tablespoon lemon juice

½ teaspoon onion powder

½ teaspoon garlic powder

½ teaspoon freshly ground black pepper

½ teaspoon salt (optional)

In the bowl of a food processor or in a blender jar, place the yeast, water, olive oil, miso, tahini, sage, lemon juice, onion powder, garlic powder, pepper, and salt, if using, and blend until smooth.

MAKES 1½ CUPS

⪗ Faux Bleu Cheese Dressing ⪖

½ cup tahini

½ cup olive oil

¼ cup lemon juice

¼ cup white vinegar

1 tablespoon finely chopped fresh
   parsley

1 teaspoon garlic powder

1 teaspoon chickpea miso

1½ teaspoons salt

1 teaspoon freshly ground black pepper

1 cup water

In the bowl of a food processor or in a blender jar, place the tahini, olive oil, lemon juice, vinegar, parsley, garlic powder, miso, salt, pepper, and water and blend until smooth.

MAKES 2½ CUPS

⪗ Balsamic Vinaigrette ⪖

1 cup olive oil

½ cup balsamic vinegar

½ teaspoon salt

¼ teaspoon freshly ground black
   pepper

⅛ teaspoon mustard seeds

In the bowl of a food processor or in a blender jar, place the olive oil, vinegar, salt, pepper, and mustard seeds and blend until smooth, or, in a small mixing bowl, whisk all of the ingredients together by hand until well blended.

MAKES 1½ CUPS

⇝ Caesar Dressing ⇜

½ cup olive oil

2 teaspoons fresh lemon juice

4 tablespoons vegan mayonnaise

1 teaspoon Dijon mustard

2 teaspoons nutritional yeast

1 teaspoon vegan Worcestershire sauce

2 teaspoons capers (with brine)

2 large cloves garlic, finely chopped

½ teaspoon salt

½ teaspoon freshly ground black
pepper

In the bowl of a food processor or in a blender jar, place the olive oil, lemon juice, mayonnaise, mustard, nutritional yeast, Worcestershire sauce, capers, garlic, salt, and pepper and blend well, or, in a small mixing bowl, whisk all of the ingredients together by hand until well blended.

MAKES 1 CUP

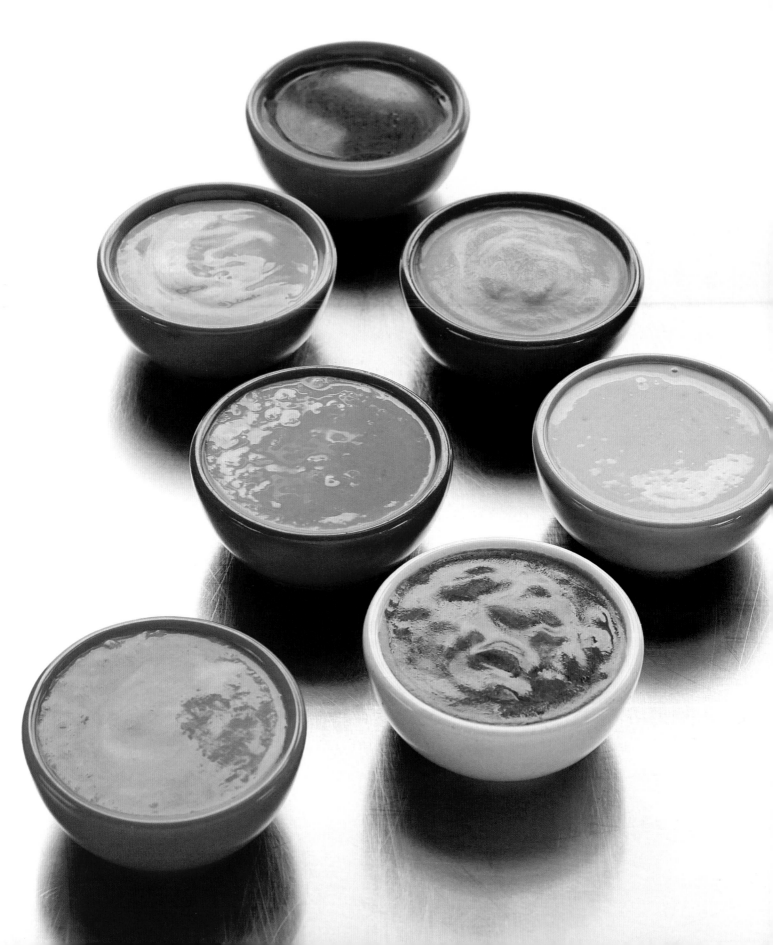

❧ Mustard Dressing ☙

1 cup olive oil

1 yellow onion, diced

½ cup brown rice vinegar

½ cup Dijon mustard

2 tablespoons agave

1 teaspoon paprika

¼ teaspoon cayenne pepper

½ teaspoon salt

¼ teaspoon freshly ground black
pepper

In the bowl of a food processor or in a blender jar, place the olive oil, onion, vinegar, mustard, agave, paprika, cayenne, salt, and pepper and blend until smooth, or place all of the ingredients in a deep bowl and blend with an immersion blender.

MAKES 2¼ CUPS

❧ Turmeric-Tahini Dressing ☙

1 cup olive oil

½ cup lemon juice

½ cup tahini

¾ cup water

1 teaspoon turmeric powder

1 teaspoon salt

½ cup finely chopped fresh parsley

In the bowl of a food processor or in a blender jar, place the olive oil, lemon juice, tahini, water, turmeric, and salt and blend until smooth. Add the parsley and blend just a second or two more, until all of the ingredients are combined. Do not overblend or the dressing will turn green!

MAKES 2¾ CUPS

⮑ Chimichurri Sauce ⮐

2 cups chopped fresh parsley

½ cup chopped fresh cilantro

1 cup olive oil

½ cup lemon juice

4 cloves garlic

1½ teaspoons cumin

1 teaspoon salt

½ teaspoon cayenne pepper

In the bowl of a food processor or in a blender jar, place the parsley, cilantro, olive oil, lemon juice, garlic, cumin, salt, and cayenne and blend until smooth, or, in a small mixing bowl, whisk all of the ingredients together by hand until well blended.

MAKES 1½ CUPS

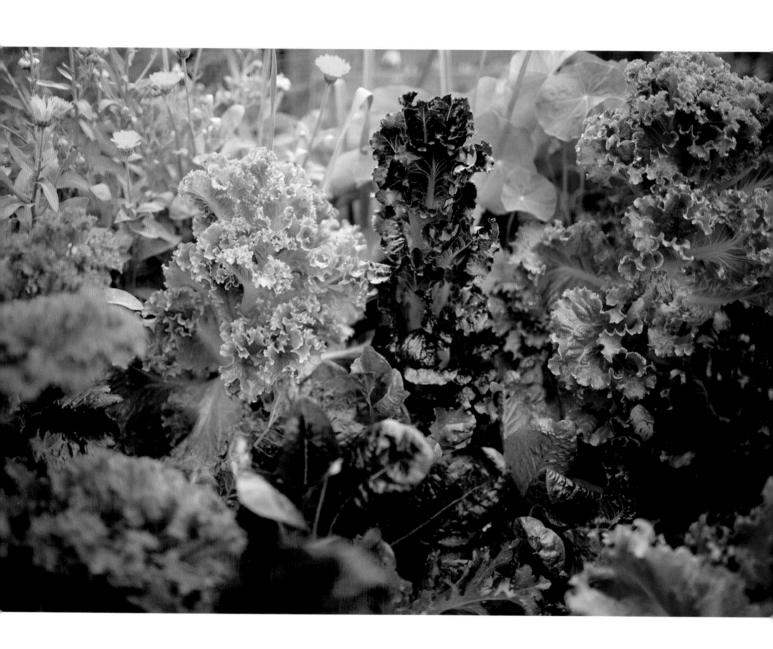

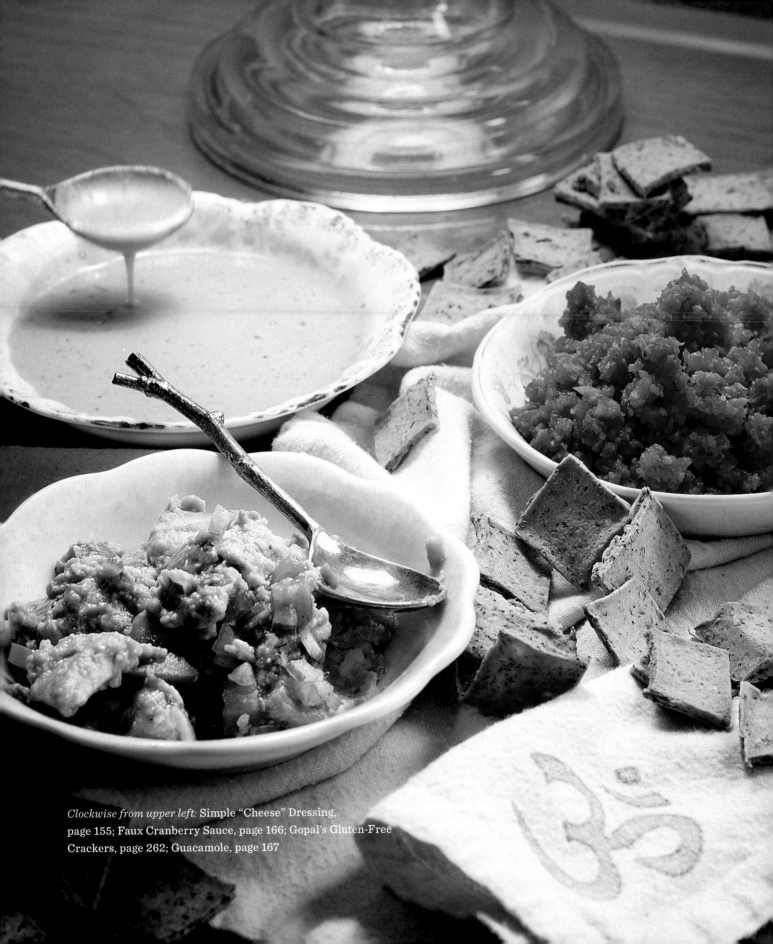

Clockwise from upper left: Simple "Cheese" Dressing,
page 155; Faux Cranberry Sauce, page 166; Gopal's Gluten-Free
Crackers, page 262; Guacamole, page 167

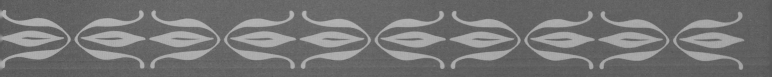

Dips and Spreads

Delectable concoctions for bread, crackers, or vegetables.

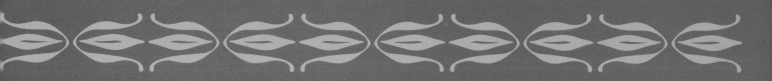

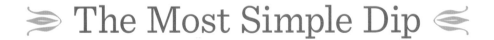 The Most Simple Dip

1 clove garlic, finely chopped

1 tablespoon dried rosemary

½ cup olive oil

In a shallow dish, place the garlic and rosemary and mix well. Pour the olive oil over the mixture and stir to combine.

MAKES ½ CUP

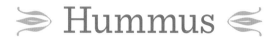

Hummus

I developed this recipe with Touria, Jivamuktea Café's magnificent, Moroccan-born chef.

1 cup dried chickpeas

3 cups water, plus more for soaking

One 1-inch piece dried kombu seaweed

1 bay leaf

1 small onion, chopped

3 cloves garlic, chopped

1 teaspoon ground cumin

½ cup tahini

3 tablespoons lemon juice

2 tablespoons olive oil

1 tablespoon paprika

1½ teaspoons salt

1½ teaspoons freshly ground black
   pepper

In a large pot, place the chickpeas and add enough water to cover by 1 inch, then soak overnight.

Drain the chickpeas and return them to the pot. Add the 3 cups water, kombu, bay leaf, onion, garlic, and cumin. Cover and bring to a boil over high heat. Reduce the heat to medium-low and cook, stirring occasionally, for about 2 hours, or until the chickpeas are fully tender. Remove from the heat and drain, reserving the cooking liquid. Discard the bay leaf. Allow the chickpeas and liquid to cool.

In the bowl of a food processor, place the cooled chickpeas, tahini, lemon juice, olive oil, paprika, salt, and pepper and blend, adding cooking liquid as necessary to yield a smooth and creamy texture.

MAKES 2 CUPS

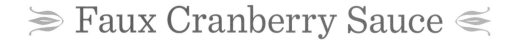 Faux Cranberry Sauce

Why "faux" cranberry sauce? Because cranberries are seasonal, but with this recipe, you can enjoy the tart wonder of cranberry sauce any time of year.

1 carrot, peeled and coarsely chopped

1 beet, peeled and coarsely chopped

1 apple, cored and coarsely chopped

One ½-inch piece fresh ginger, peeled and coarsely chopped

1 tablespoon lemon juice

In the bowl of a food processor or in a blender jar, place the carrot, beet, apple, ginger, and lemon juice and blend. Do not add water; the consistency should remain chunky, resembling cranberry sauce in texture and taste. Serve as you would cranberry sauce (but without the turkey, of course!).

MAKES 1 CUP

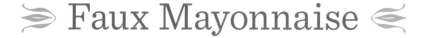 Faux Mayonnaise

Commercially prepared vegan mayonnaise does exist, but I prefer this homemade version because it is fresh, low in fat, and free of preservatives and stabilizers.

8 ounces soft tofu

1 tablespoon almond butter

2 tablespoons lemon juice

2 tablespoons agave

1 clove garlic, chopped

½ teaspoon salt

In the bowl of a food processor or in a blender jar, place the tofu, almond butter, lemon juice, agave, garlic, and salt and blend until smooth and creamy.

MAKES 1 CUP

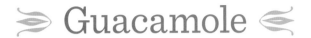 Guacamole

Guacamole makes a surprisingly good side dish on its own. It's not just for chips anymore!

2 ripe avocados, peeled and pits removed

1 tomato, chopped into small pieces

2 tablespoons finely chopped red onion

2 tablespoons commercially prepared green chili sauce

1 tablespoon lime juice

Salt to taste

In a small bowl, place the avocados and mash them with a fork. Add the tomato, onion, chili sauce, lime juice, and salt to taste and mix well.

MAKES 1½ CUPS

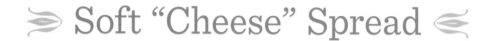 Soft "Cheese" Spread

Julia Butterfly, the well-known activist, was visiting me in Woodstock once, and we put our heads together to come up with a way to make a simple vegan cheese. This spread was the result.

½ cup nutritional yeast flakes

½ cup pastry flour

1 teaspoon salt

1 teaspoon turmeric powder

½ teaspoon garlic powder

1½ cups water, plus more as needed

4 tablespoons (½ stick) vegan
    margarine

1 teaspoon prepared mustard

In a small saucepan, place the nutritional yeast, flour, salt, turmeric, and garlic powder and, using a fork or a wire whisk, slowly whisk in the water. When combined, cook over medium heat, continuing to whisk, until the mixture thickens and bubbles. Cook for 30 more seconds then remove from heat. Using a large spoon, whip in the margarine and mustard. The spread will thicken as it cools, so add more water to thin it, if necessary.

MAKES 1½ CUPS

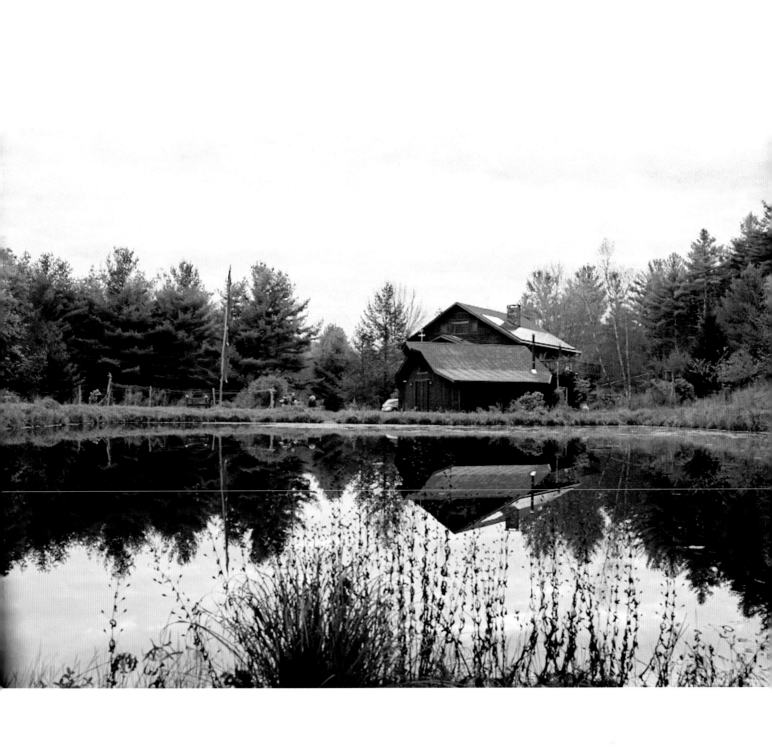

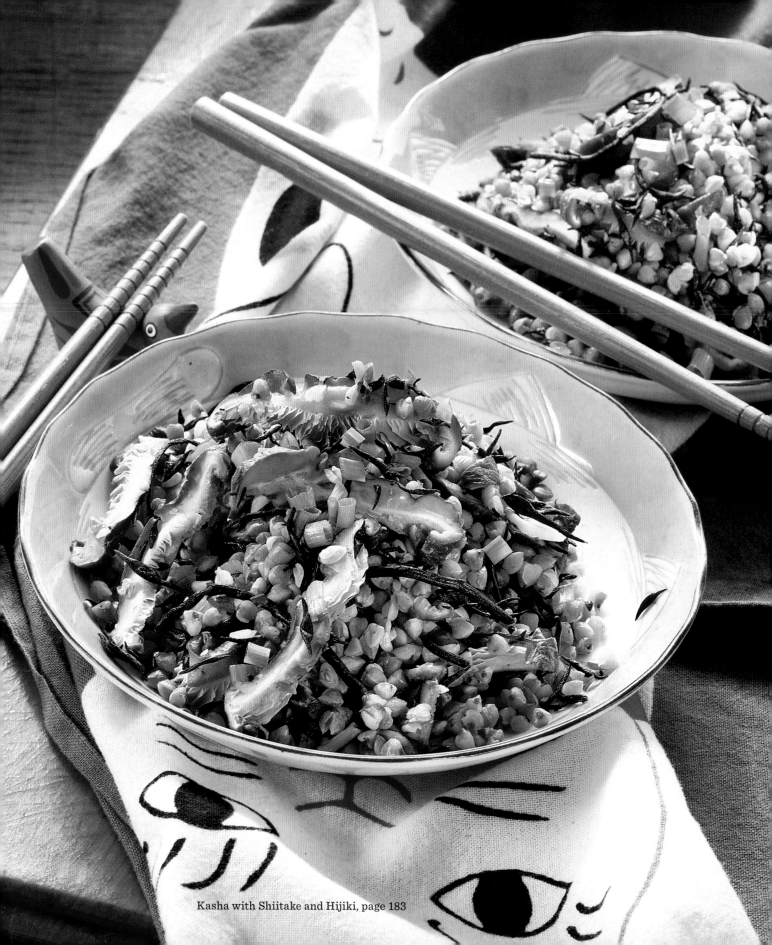

Kasha with Shiitake and Hijiki, page 183

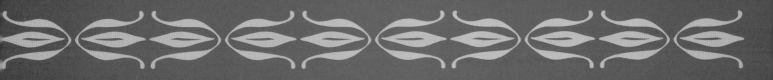

Grains

Grains are the dried seeds from cereals like rice, wheat, millet, quinoa, corn, and kasha. They can be whole, with the outer shell of the seed kernel left intact, or polished/processed, with the outer shell removed. Grains can be prepared in many ways, as well as ground into flour for breads and crackers. Grains provide complex carbohydrates, fiber, fats, proteins, and many vitamins and minerals, making them an important staple for human beings for thousands of years.

The basic recipe for cooking most whole grains is to use one part grain to two parts water, place in a pot with a tight-fitting lid, bring to a boil, then reduce the heat to low and simmer until the water is absorbed. Cooking times differ for different grains: brown rice takes about 40 minutes, while white rice, quinoa, kasha, and most other grains take about 20 minutes. The rest of this chapter has specialty recipes using various types of grains. When the recipe calls for cooked grains, they should be cooked using this basic recipe.

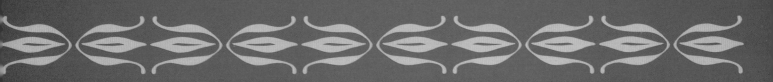

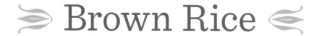 Brown Rice

1 cup short-grain brown rice
2 cups water

In a medium pot, place the rice and water, cover, and bring to a boil over high heat. Stir a few times, then cover with a tight-fitting lid, reduce the heat to low, and simmer for about 40 minutes, or until steam holes appear in the rice. Remove from the heat, fluff with a fork, and serve immediately.

SERVES 2 TO 4

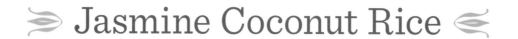 Jasmine Coconut Rice

This rice pairs nicely with Asian-inspired dishes but is also great on its own.

2 cups cooked jasmine rice
One 10- to 15-ounce can coconut milk
1 tablespoon agave

½ cup dried shredded nori or tamari-
flavored seaweed

In a medium bowl, place the rice, coconut milk, agave, and seaweed and mix well.

SERVES 2 TO 4

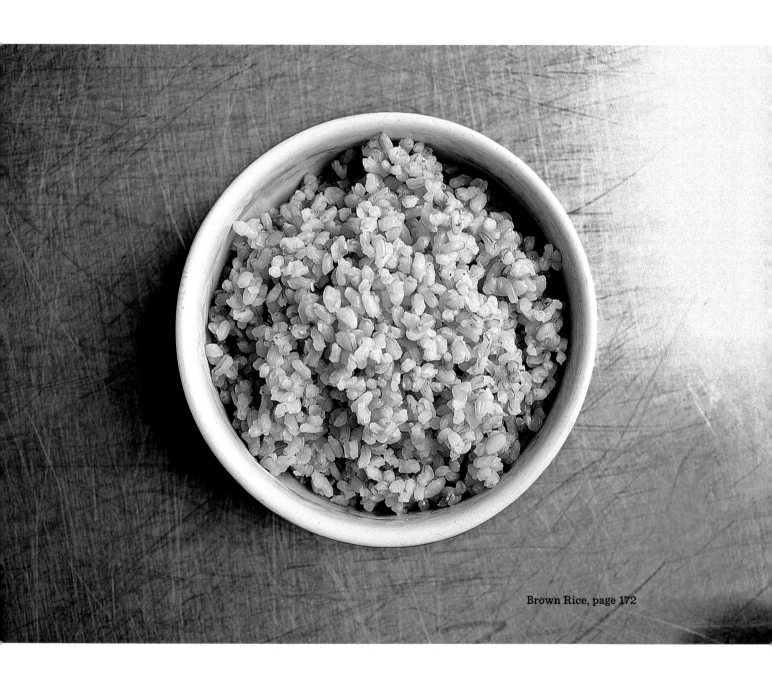

Brown Rice, page 172

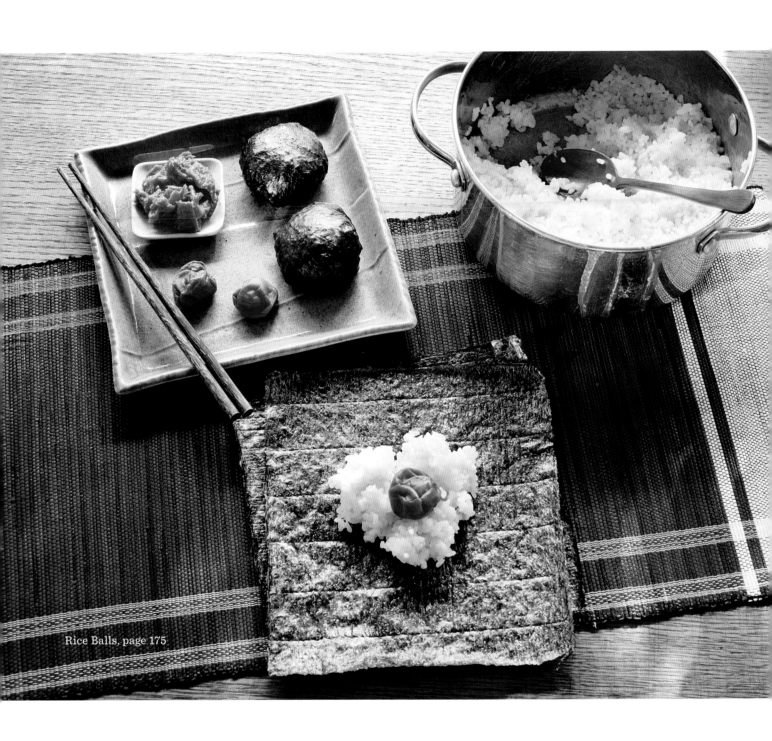

Rice Balls, page 175

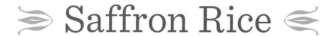 Saffron Rice

I use sticky rice for this recipe, but any kind of white rice will do well. Iranian saffron is stronger and more expensive than Turkish saffron, but you don't need as much.

1 cup uncooked white sticky rice
1 tablespoon Turkish saffron, or
   1 teaspoon Iranian saffron

½ cup fresh or frozen peas
2 cups water

In a medium saucepan, place the rice, saffron, peas, and water, bring to a boil over high heat, cover, reduce the heat to low, and cook for 20 minutes.

SERVES 2 TO 4

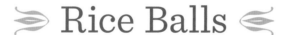 Rice Balls

A simple lunch or satisfying snack, rice balls are very popular in Japan. Whenever I bite into one of these delicacies, I'm always pleasantly surprised to discover the plum treasure waiting inside.

2 cups cooked white sticky rice
8 sheets toasted nori

8 umeboshi plums, pitted, or equivalent
   in umeboshi paste

Using wet hands, divide the rice into 8 balls. Place one ball of rice on each nori sheet, shiny side down, insert a plum into the center (or spread a bit of umeboshi paste on the rice), then fold the nori around the rice. Wet the edges of the nori to help it stick together.

MAKES 8 RICE BALLS

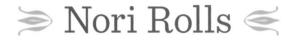 Nori Rolls

The credit for this recipe really goes to Julie Kirkpatrick, who is one mean nori roller. Over the years I think she has rolled thousands of these for our Fourth of July celebrations in Woodstock.

1 large carrot, peeled and cut into
   6 long thin strips

1 teaspoon wasabi powder

1 tablespoon lemon juice

3 tablespoons mirin

2 teaspoons sugar

1 teaspoon salt

2 cups cooked white sticky rice, cooled
   to room temperature

6 sheets toasted nori

½ avocado, cut into thin strips

1 cucumber, peeled and cut into
   6 long strips

Soy sauce, tamari, or Braggs Liquid
   Aminos

In a steamer basket set over boiling water, place the carrot strips and steam them until almost but not quite soft, 5 to 8 minutes.

In a small bowl, mix the wasabi powder with a little water to make a paste and set aside. In a small cup, place the lemon juice, mirin, sugar, and salt and add just enough boiling water to dissolve the sugar and salt. Stir well, place the rice in a large bowl, pour in the lemon mixture, and mix well.

On a cutting board or bamboo sushi mat, place 1 sheet of nori, shiny side down. Wet your hands and, using a ⅓-cup measuring cup, scoop about ⅓ cup of rice onto each sheet, spreading it out but leaving a 1-inch border on the far and near sides. In the middle of the rice, press a slice of avocado, a slice of cucumber, and a slice of carrot. Starting with the side closest to you, begin to roll the sheet into a long cylinder and set aside. Do the same until all of the rolls are made. Finally, using a very sharp knife, cut the rolls crosswise. It is helpful to make your first cut in the center, dividing the cylinder in half, and then slicing each half in thirds. Each roll should yield 6 bite-size nori rolls.

To make a dipping sauce, add soy sauce to the wasabi paste until the sauce is thin.

MAKES 36 ROLLS

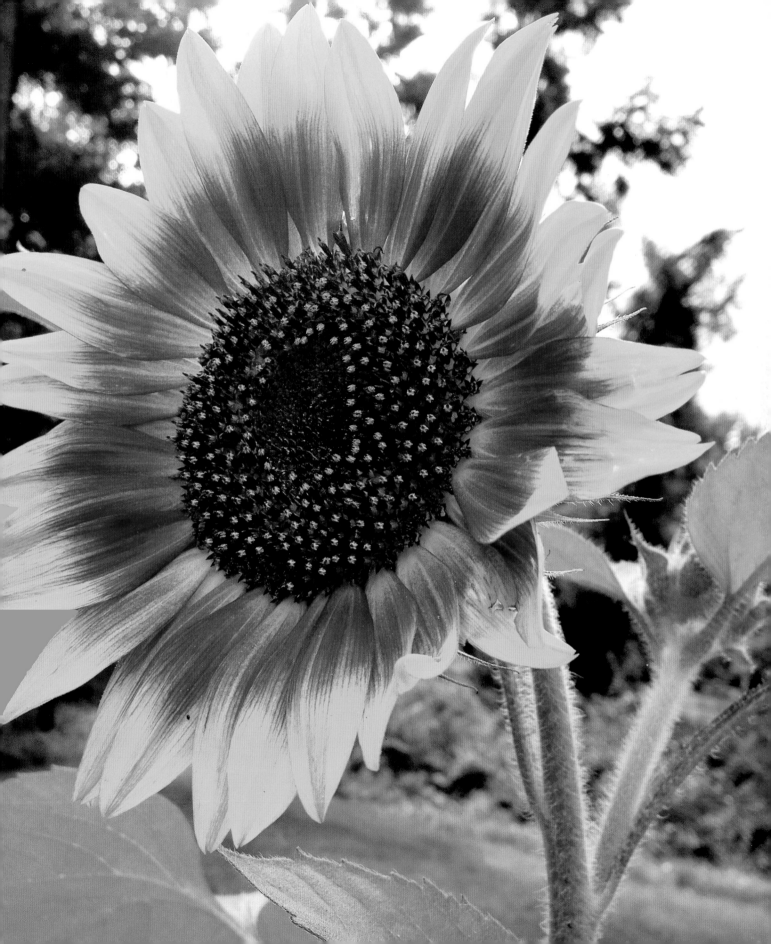

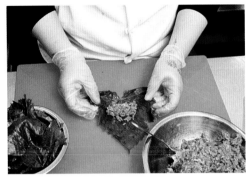

1.

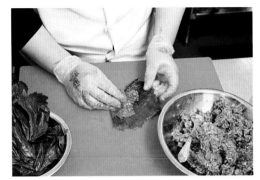

2.

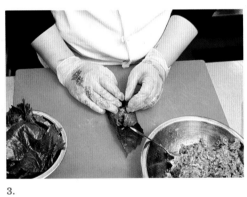

3.

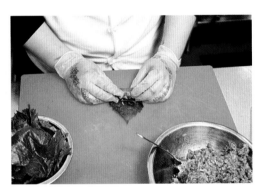

4.

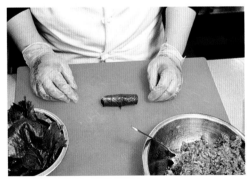

5.

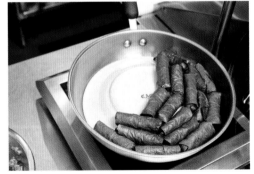

6.

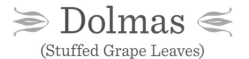

Dolmas

(Stuffed Grape Leaves)

The trick to making dolmas is in the folding and rolling.

1 tablespoon olive oil

2 onions, finely chopped

1½ cups uncooked white rice

2 tablespoons tomato paste

2 tablespoons dried currants or raisins

1 teaspoon ground cinnamon

1 teaspoon dried mint

1 teaspoon dried dill weed

1 teaspoon ground allspice

1 teaspoon ground cumin

One 8-ounce jar grape leaves, drained

In a medium saucepan, heat the olive oil over medium heat. Add the onions and sauté for about 10 minutes, until tender. Stir in the rice and just enough hot water to cover. Reduce the heat to low, cover the pan, and simmer until the rice is half cooked, about 10 minutes. Remove from the heat and stir in the tomato paste, currants, cinnamon, mint, dill, allspice, and cumin. Let the mixture cool.

Prepare a large pot by placing an inverted heatproof plate on the bottom; this is to protect the dolmas from direct heat when steaming. Rinse the grape leaves in warm water, drain, and cut off any stems. Place about 1 teaspoon of the cooled rice mixture in the center of a leaf. Fold in the sides and then roll into a cigar-like cylinder shape. Place the dolma in the prepared pot. Repeat with remaining leaves and rice mixture. Pour just enough warm water in the pot to reach the bottom of the first layer of dolmas. Steam the dolmas for about 10 minutes, checking the water level often and adding more as necessary.

MAKES 40 DOLMAS

MILLET

⇒ Spirulina Millet ⇐

This is Jivamuktea Café's signature dish. You won't find this at any other restaurant because I developed it in my own kitchen and have been serving it to dinner guests—including my cats—for about thirty years. It has everything—protein, omega-3 fatty acids, chlorophyll, and, of course, incredible taste! It's great as a side dish and even as a spread on toast, where the taste evokes an aged cheese. I like to use a fork to mix all of the ingredients, but some people might prefer to use their hands.

1 cup uncooked millet

2 cups water

¼ cup flaxseed oil

¼ cup powdered spirulina

1 tablespoon soy sauce, tamari, or
  Braggs Liquid Aminos

In a medium pot, place the millet and water, cover, and bring to a boil over high heat. Reduce the heat to low and simmer for about 20 minutes, until the liquid is absorbed. Turn off heat and let the millet sit uncovered after cooking for about 10 minutes so it dries out some, then transfer it to a large bowl. Add the flaxseed oil and, using a large fork, mix well to coat the millet. Little by little, add the spirulina, using the fork to mix. Add the soy sauce, mixing well until the millet is bright green.

SERVES 4 TO 6

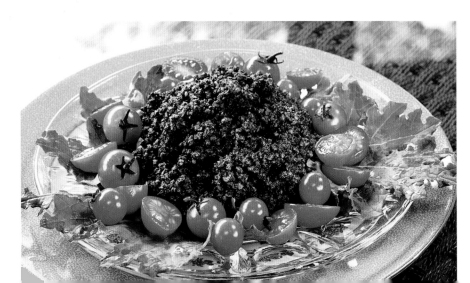

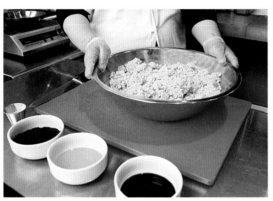

1.

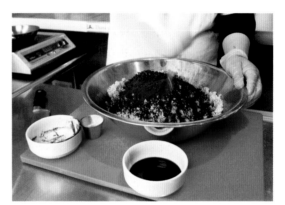

2.

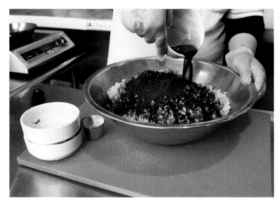

3.

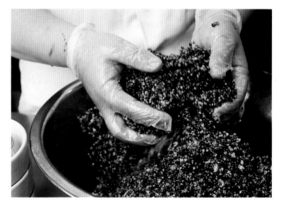

4.

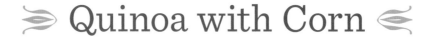 Quinoa with Corn

1 cup uncooked quinoa
1 cup fresh or frozen corn
2¼ cups water

In a medium saucepan, place the quinoa, corn, and water and bring to a boil over high heat. Reduce the heat to low and simmer, covered, for 20 minutes. Turn off the heat and let sit, covered, for about 5 minutes, until the quinoa is fully expanded and tender.

SERVES 2 TO 4

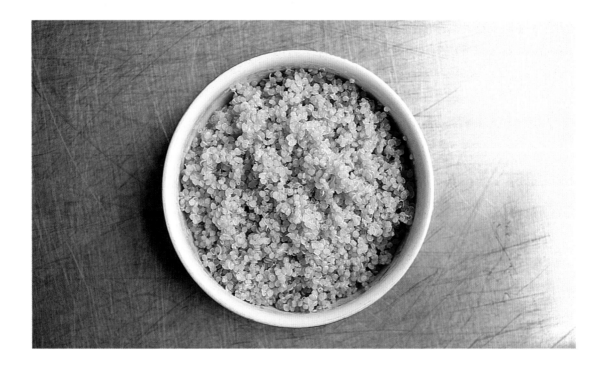

⮵ Kasha with ⮶ Shiitake and Hijiki

5 dried shiitake mushrooms

¼ cup dried hijiki seaweed

1 cup uncooked kasha

In a small bowl, place the mushrooms and seaweed. Add boiling water to cover and let stand for 5 to 10 minutes to rehydrate. Drain, and reserve the soaking water. Using kitchen scissors, cut the mushrooms into very thin strips.

In a small saucepan, place the mushrooms, seaweed, and kasha. Pour the reserved soaking water into a measuring cup and top off with enough water to make 2 cups of liquid. Pour the liquid into the saucepan, cover, and bring to a boil over high heat. Turn off the heat and let the kasha sit for about 10 minutes, until all of the water is absorbed.

SERVES 2 TO 4

≽ Kasha with ≼ Black-Eyed Peas

One 15-ounce can black-eyed peas, with liquid

1 cup uncooked kasha

2 tablespoons finely chopped red onion

1½ cups water

1 tablespoon toasted sesame oil

½ cup grated commercially prepared vegan cheese

8 to 10 tortilla chips, broken into small pieces

1 tablespoon soy sauce, tamari, or Braggs Liquid Aminos

In a medium saucepan, place the black-eyed peas, kasha, onions, water, and sesame oil. Cover and bring to a boil over high heat. Remove the cover, stir in the cheese, chips, and soy sauce, turn off the heat, and let sit for about 10 minutes.

SERVES 2 TO 4

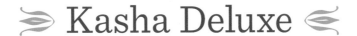 Kasha Deluxe

2 tablespoons sunflower oil

8 ounces mushrooms (any type), sliced

½ onion, finely chopped

4 ounces firm tofu, cubed

One 4-inch sprig fresh rosemary, finely
chopped, or 1 tablespoon dried
rosemary

4 cloves garlic, finely chopped

2 cups cooked kasha

¼ cup hulled sunflower seeds

Salt and freshly ground black pepper
to taste

In a large frying pan, heat the sunflower oil over medium-high heat. Add the mushrooms, onion, tofu, rosemary, and garlic and sauté for 5 to 10 minutes, until the onions are translucent. Stir in the kasha and sunflower seeds, and add salt and pepper to taste.

SERVES 4 TO 6

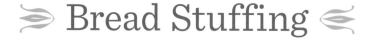

Bread Stuffing

Traditionally, bread stuffing is used to stuff a turkey or chicken. But usually at holiday dinners, even meat eaters say it's not the bird that's the hit, it's the stuffing. So why not just eat the stuffing and leave the bird off the menu altogether?

½ cup dried mushrooms, any variety, cut into small pieces

1 tablespoon powdered vegetable stock or equivalent in bouillon cubes

1½ cups boiling water

2 tablespoons olive oil

1 cup walnuts

6 tablespoons (¾ stick) vegan margarine

1 loaf very dry day-old bread, any kind, cut into ¾-inch cubes (about 10 cups)

1 cup chopped onion

1 cup chopped celery

1 apple, cored and chopped into ½-inch pieces

¾ cup raisins

¼ cup chopped fresh parsley

2 teaspoons ground sage

Salt and freshly ground black pepper to taste

In a small bowl, place the mushrooms, stock, and water and set aside for 5 to 10 minutes, to rehydrate.

In a medium frying pan, heat the olive oil over medium-high heat. Add the walnuts and toast for about 3 minutes, stirring frequently, until they are slightly browned, taking care not to let them burn. Lay the nuts in a single layer on a brown paper bag to drain and cool. When cooled, coarsely chop the walnuts into small pieces and set aside.

In a large cast-iron Dutch oven, melt 3 tablespoons of the margarine over medium heat. Add the bread cubes, stirring to coat, then let them toast, turning them often to brown on all sides, for 5 to 7 minutes. In a frying pan, heat the remaining 3 tablespoons margarine over medium-high heat. Add the onions and celery and sauté for 5 to 10 minutes, until the onions are translucent. To the Dutch oven, add the sautéed mixture, the mushrooms (with the soaking liquid), walnuts, apple, raisins, parsley, sage, and salt and pepper to taste and mix thoroughly. Reduce the heat to low, cover the pot, and cook for 1 hour. Check every 10 minutes or so. Stir the stuffing and add water as needed to keep the stuffing moist and to prevent it from sticking to the bottom of the pan.

SERVES 6 TO 8

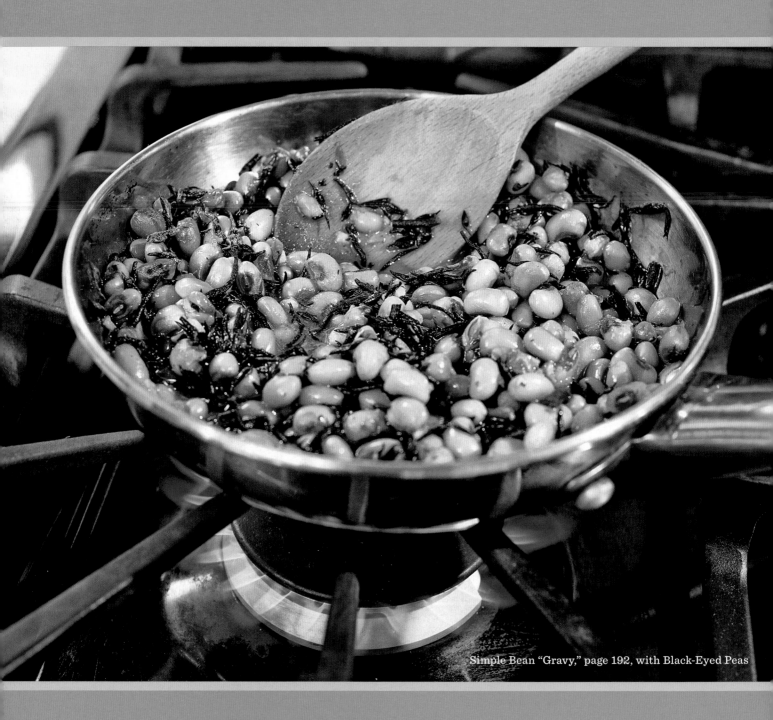

Simple Bean "Gravy," page 192, with Black-Eyed Peas

Beans, Tempeh, Tofu, and Seitan

Although it is true that all vegetables contain protein, wheat gluten, beans, and bean products (like tempeh and tofu) contain higher amounts of protein than most vegetables. Even though it is not necessary to serve beans with grains to obtain the minimum daily requirement of protein, beans and grains complement each other in taste and texture.

Want to know a tip for counteracting the gas-producing effects of beans? Cook them with a small amount of seaweed!

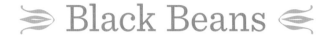 Black Beans

Smooth, savory, and satisfying to the most discriminating of palates.

2 cups dried black beans

10 cups water

One 1-inch piece dried kombu seaweed

2 bay leaves

2 tablespoons (¼ stick) vegan
  margarine

2 tablespoons ground cumin

1 tablespoon salt

In a large bowl or pot, place the beans, add 6 cups of the water, and soak overnight.

Drain the beans and transfer them to a pot with the remaining 4 cups water. Add the kombu, bay leaves, margarine, and cumin, and bring to a boil, covered, over high heat. Reduce the heat to medium-high and cook, covered, stirring occasionally, for about 2 hours, or until the beans are fully tender. Remove from the heat, add the salt, and stir well. Discard the bay leaves. The beans can be stored in a tightly sealed container in the refrigerator for up to 5 days.

SERVES 8 TO 10

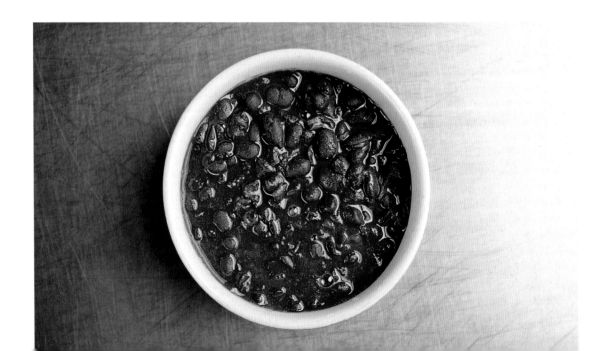

⇒ Smoky Pinto Beans ⇐

This recipe lends a slightly smoky taste to the beans, as if cooked over a campfire.

2 cups dried pinto beans

11 cups water

One 1-inch piece dried kombu seaweed

2 bay leaves

½ onion, finely chopped

4 cloves garlic, finely chopped

2 tablespoons ground cumin

½ tablespoon red pepper flakes

½ teaspoon vegan liquid smoke

1 tablespoon salt

In a large bowl or pot, place the beans, add 6 cups of the water, and soak overnight.

Drain the beans and transfer them to a pot with the remaining 5 cups water. Add the kombu, bay leaves, onion, garlic, cumin, red pepper flakes, and liquid smoke and bring to a boil, covered, over high heat. Reduce the heat to medium-high and cook, covered, stirring occasionally, for about 2 hours, or until the beans are fully tender. Remove from the heat, add the salt, and stir well. Discard the bay leaves. The beans can be stored in a tightly sealed container in the refrigerator for up to 5 days.

SERVES 8 TO 10

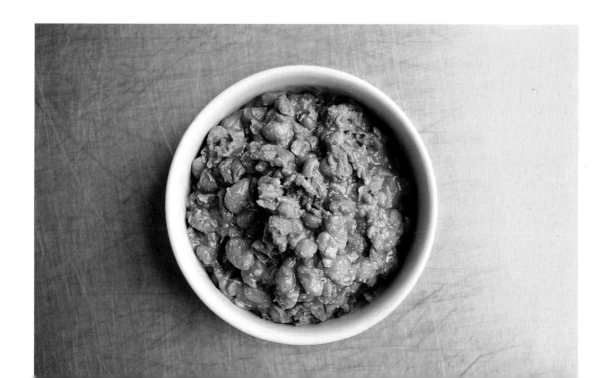

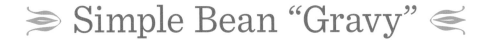 Simple Bean "Gravy"

This is my signature bean recipe. I call it "gravy" because the beans become
sauce-like and lend themselves to being poured over mashed potatoes, rice,
or any other grain—or eaten as they are as a side dish, with a spoon!

1 tablespoon dried hijiki seaweed
½ cup boiling water
One 15-ounce can beans, any kind, with
   their liquid

1 teaspoon soy sauce, tamari, or Braggs
   Liquid Aminos

In a small saucepan, place the seaweed, add the water, and simmer over low heat for about 5 minutes. Pour the beans with their liquid into the saucepan and cook, covered, over low heat for about 5 minutes. Add the soy sauce. For a creamier, smoother gravy, blend with an immersion blender before serving.

SERVES 2 TO 4

⇒ Deluxe White Bean ⇐ "Gravy"

This gravy tastes so rich and creamy, everyone is surprised that it is almost fat-free.

5 fresh or dried mushrooms, any kind
1 tablespoon dried hijiki seaweed
2 tablespoons olive oil
½ red onion, finely chopped
4 cloves garlic, finely chopped
1 sprig fresh tarragon, or 1 tablespoon
    dried tarragon

One 15-ounce can cannellini beans, with
    their liquid
1 tablespoon lemon juice
Salt and freshly ground black pepper
    to taste

If using dried mushrooms, in a small bowl place the dried mushrooms and the seaweed, add boiling water to cover, and let stand for 5 to 10 minutes to rehydrate. If using fresh mushrooms, then just rehydrate the seaweed. Drain the rehydrated mushrooms and/or seaweed and reserve the soaking liquid. Slice the mushrooms into thin strips.

In a large frying pan, heat the olive oil over medium heat. Add the mushrooms, onion, garlic, and tarragon and sauté for 5 to 10 minutes, until the onions are translucent. Add the seaweed, beans, and reserved soaking liquid, cover, and bring to a boil over high heat. Reduce the heat to low and simmer for about 10 minutes. Add a little more water, if needed, to obtain the desired consistency. Add the lemon juice and salt and pepper to taste. For a creamier gravy, blend with an immersion blender before serving.

SERVES 2 TO 4

⇌ Sweet and Crunchy ⇌ Rice and Beans

I've taken the traditional marriage of rice and beans and created contrasting pairs of sweet and savory, raw and cooked, and smooth and crunchy to make this dish a passionate love affair.

2 tablespoons dried hijiki seaweed

One 15-ounce can adzuki beans, with their liquid

4 cloves garlic, finely chopped

1 teaspoon red pepper flakes

2 tablespoons agave or maple syrup

2 tablespoons rice vinegar

1 tablespoon toasted sesame oil

1 tablespoon soy sauce, tamari, or Braggs Liquid Aminos

1 cup cooked brown rice

12 ounces raw mung bean sprouts

¼ red onion, diced

2 scallions, chopped

2 cups broken corn chips

In a small bowl, place the seaweed, add boiling water to cover, and let stand for 5 minutes to rehydrate.

Place the beans in a medium saucepan. Add the garlic and red pepper flakes and cook, covered, over medium heat for 10 minutes. Reduce the heat to low, add the agave, vinegar, sesame oil, and soy sauce. Stir well, remove from the heat, and set aside.

Place the rice, sprouts, onion, and scallions in a large bowl and mix well. Add the bean mixture and stir together, then sprinkle with the corn chips.

SERVES 2 TO 4

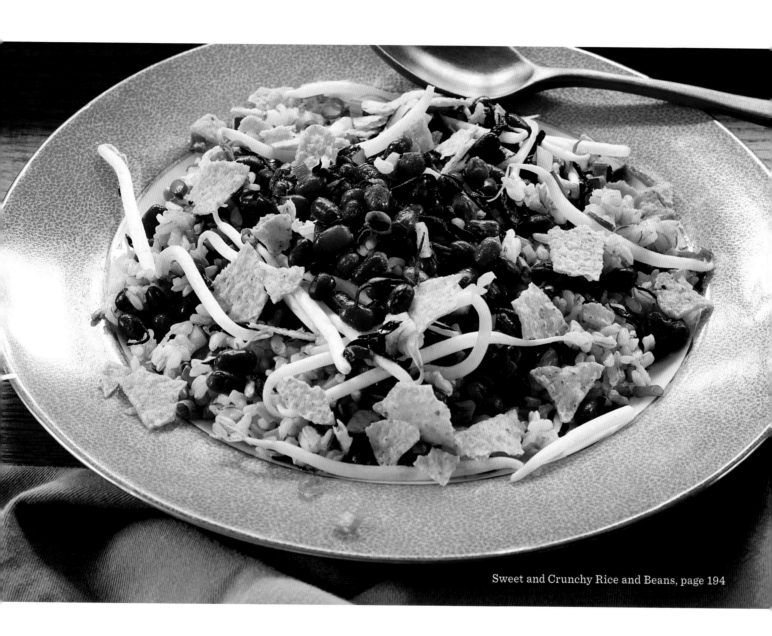

Sweet and Crunchy Rice and Beans, page 194

⋟ Beans and Faux Chicken ⋞

This is quick and simple to make, and oh so tasty!

¼ cup olive oil

3 cloves garlic, finely chopped

1 tablespoon fresh oregano, or
1 teaspoon dried oregano

1 package commercially prepared
"chicken-style" seitan, cut into small,
thin strips

One 15-ounce can garbanzo beans,
liquid drained

Salt and freshly ground black pepper
to taste

In a medium frying pan, heat the olive oil over medium heat. Add the garlic, oregano, and seitan and sauté for 3 minutes, then add the beans and cook for another minute. Reduce the heat to low and simmer for 5 minutes, then add salt and pepper to taste.

SERVES 2 TO 4

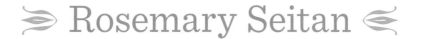 Rosemary Seitan

The addition of mustard and mayonnaise results in an irresistible,
stroganoff-like consistency, but without the cream.

¼ cup safflower oil or olive oil

1 pound seitan, cut into thin strips

¼ cup dried cranberries

½ cup diced celery

¼ cup kalamata olives, thinly sliced

1 tablespoon dried rosemary

3 tablespoons Dijon mustard

3 tablespoons vegan mayonnaise

In a large frying pan, heat the safflower oil over medium heat. Add the seitan and sauté for 2 minutes. Add the cranberries, celery, olives, and rosemary and cook for 3 to 5 minutes, stirring often and adding a bit of water if necessary to keep the mixture from sticking, until well mixed and well heated. Add the mustard and mayonnaise and mix well.

SERVES 2 TO 4

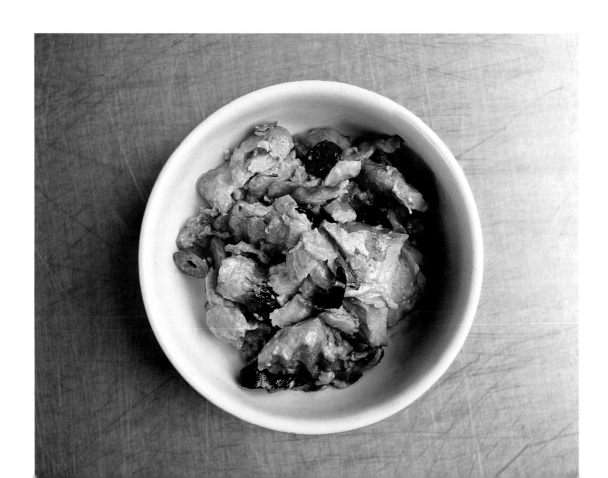

⇌ French Tarragon, ⇋ Chanterelle, and Sausages

I must admit that even when I did eat meat, I never ate sausages. But now that I am vegan and vegan sausages—made from a variety of vegetable sources such as soybeans, wheat, and even green peas—are readily available, I have really acquired a taste for them. Perhaps I'm spoiled because faux meats are available in most health food stores in America, and I live in a forest where wild mushrooms grow, but I hope that you will be able to find all the ingredients in your local grocery store. If you can't find them, remember that these days you can order almost anything online. This dish is particularly good served with Saffron Rice (page 175).

¼ cup olive oil

6 cloves garlic, finely chopped

Four 6-inch-long commercially prepared vegan sausages or tofu hot dogs, cut into ¼-inch discs

2 tablespoons dried tarragon

1 pound chanterelle mushrooms, or any other kind, sliced

¼ cup water

Salt and freshly ground black pepper to taste

In a large frying pan, heat the olive oil over medium heat. Add the garlic, sausages, and tarragon and sauté for about 5 minutes, until the sausage is just starting to brown. Add the mushrooms and sauté for another 5 minutes. Add the water, reduce the heat to low, and simmer, covered, for another 5 minutes. Add salt and pepper to taste.

SERVES 4 TO 6

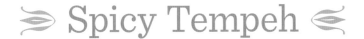 Spicy Tempeh

This is the recipe I'm asked for most often after people have tasted it at Jivamuktea Café.

½ cup safflower oil or olive oil

1 pound tempeh, cut into ½-inch cubes

1 large onion, diced

3 cloves garlic, finely chopped

1 tablespoon dried red pepper flakes

1 tablespoon dried basil

1 tablespoon dried sage

2 tablespoons soy sauce, tamari, or
    Braggs Liquid Aminos

2 tablespoons water

In a medium frying pan, heat the safflower oil. Add the tempeh and sauté for about 3 minutes, until golden brown. Add the onion, garlic, red pepper flakes, basil, and sage and stir to combine. Add the soy sauce and water and simmer, uncovered, for about 10 minutes, until well mixed and the flavors are blended.

SERVES 4 TO 6

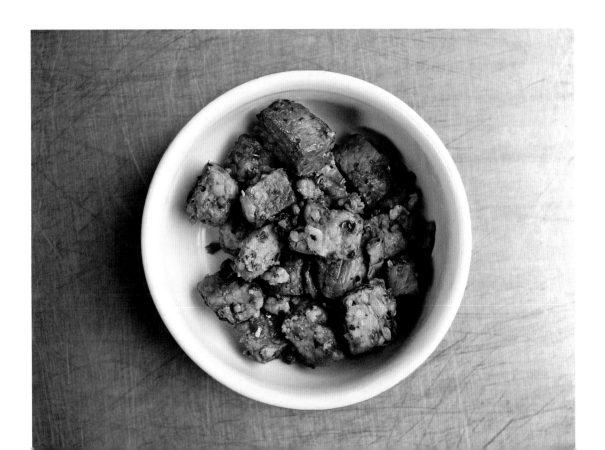

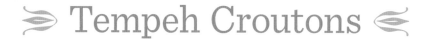 Tempeh Croutons

These croutons are great with a Caesar Salad (page 128), or with rice, kasha, or mashed potatoes, or just by themselves. For a tropical variation, substitute coconut oil for the olive oil.

¼ cup olive oil

1 pound tempeh, cut into ¼-inch cubes

¼ teaspoon salt

1 teaspoon red pepper flakes

1 teaspoon dried rosemary

In a medium frying pan, heat the olive oil over medium heat. Add the tempeh and salt and sauté for 1 to 2 minutes, turning the tempeh frequently, until it is just starting to brown. Add the red pepper flakes, and rosemary and sauté for another minute, until the tempeh is golden brown.

SERVES 4 TO 6

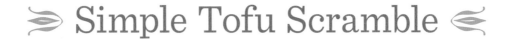 Simple Tofu Scramble

This recipe was inspired by my beloved friend Shyamdas who, as a devotee of Lord Krishna, refrained from eating garlic and onions, and certainly eggs.

1 tablespoon turmeric powder	¼ teaspoon chili powder
1 teaspoon nutritional yeast flakes	¼ teaspoon paprika
1 teaspoon ground cumin	3 tablespoons vegan margarine
½ teaspoon salt	14 ounces firm tofu, drained

In a small bowl, place the turmeric, nutritional yeast, cumin, salt, chili powder, and paprika and mix well. Add 2 to 3 tablespoons of water, just enough to make a thin liquid. Stir well, then set aside.

In a large frying pan, melt the margarine over medium heat and crumble the tofu into the pan. Sauté gently for about 1 minute, pour in the spice mixture, and stir to coat all of the tofu pieces evenly.

SERVES 2 TO 4

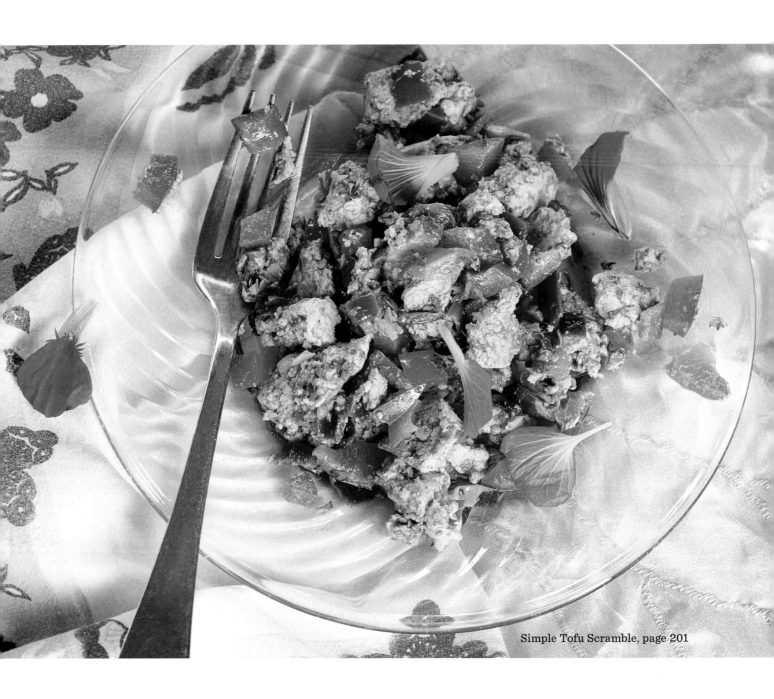

Simple Tofu Scramble, page 201

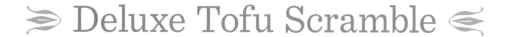 Deluxe Tofu Scramble

This tofu scramble is rapidly taking its place at the conscious breakfast table.

3 tablespoons olive oil

1 onion, chopped

1 red or green bell pepper, chopped

1 tablespoon turmeric powder

1 tablespoon nutritional yeast flakes

1 teaspoon ground cumin

1 teaspoon ground coriander

1 teaspoon dried thyme

½ teaspoon salt

¼ teaspoon paprika

¼ teaspoon chili powder

3 tablespoons vegan margarine

14 ounces firm tofu, drained

¼ cup finely chopped fresh parsley

In a large frying pan, heat the olive oil over medium heat. Add the onion and bell pepper and sauté for 5 to 10 minutes, until the onions are translucent.

Place the turmeric, nutritional yeast, cumin, coriander, thyme, salt, paprika, and chili powder in a small bowl and mix well. Add 4 to 5 tablespoons of water, just enough to make a thin liquid. Stir well and set aside.

In a large frying pan, melt the margarine over medium heat and crumble the tofu into the pan. Sauté gently for about 1 minute, then add the sautéed mixture and the spice mixture, and stir well. Cook for another 3 minutes. Just before serving, mix in the parsley.

SERVES 2 TO 4

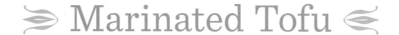

Marinated Tofu

These tasty morsels can be added to a salad or used to dress up any dish.

14 ounces firm tofu, cut into ¼-inch
   cubes
3 tablespoons soy sauce, tamari, or
   Braggs Liquid Aminos
1 tablespoon mirin

1 tablespoon agave
Salt and freshly ground black pepper
   to taste
1 scallion, chopped (optional)

In a small bowl, place the tofu cubes and add the soy sauce, mirin, and agave. Mix well, sprinkle with salt and pepper to taste, and let sit for at least 10 minutes. Garnish with scallion, if desired.

FOR A GRILLED TOFU ALTERNATIVE

Instead of cubes, slice the tofu into ¼-inch slices. Arrange the tofu slices in a shallow dish. Double the recipe for the marinade and pour over the tofu. Let sit for about 10 minutes. Arrange the tofu slices on a grill and cook for about 3 minutes, until grill marks appear on the bottom of the tofu, then turn and grill for another 3 minutes. Alternatively, broil the tofu in the oven for about the same amount of time, turning once.

SERVES 2 TO 4

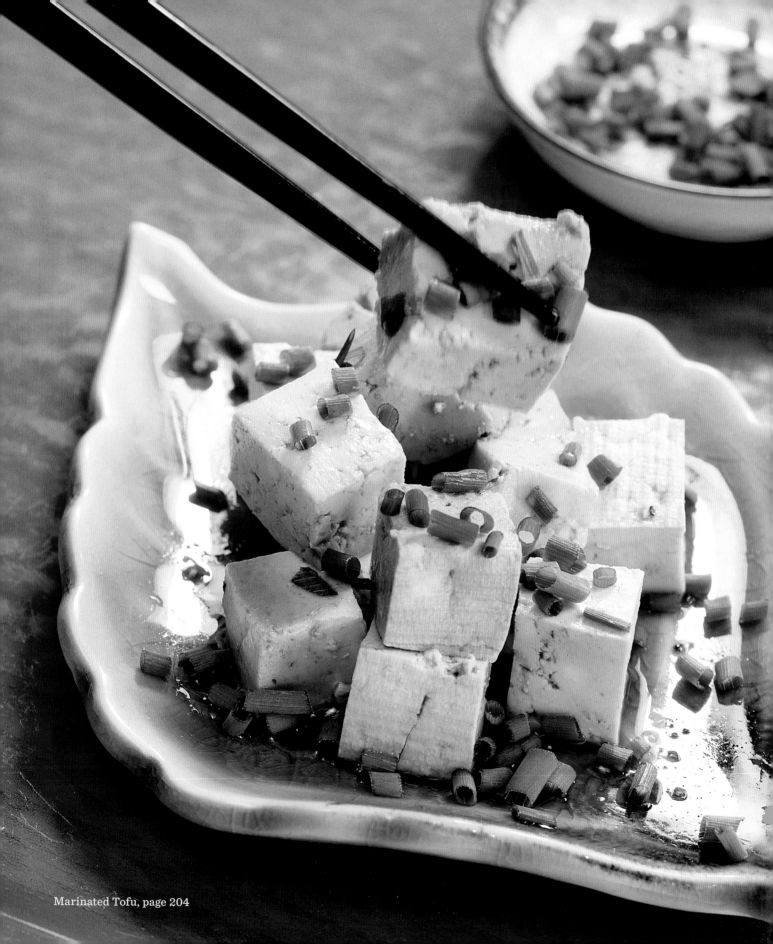

Marinated Tofu, page 204

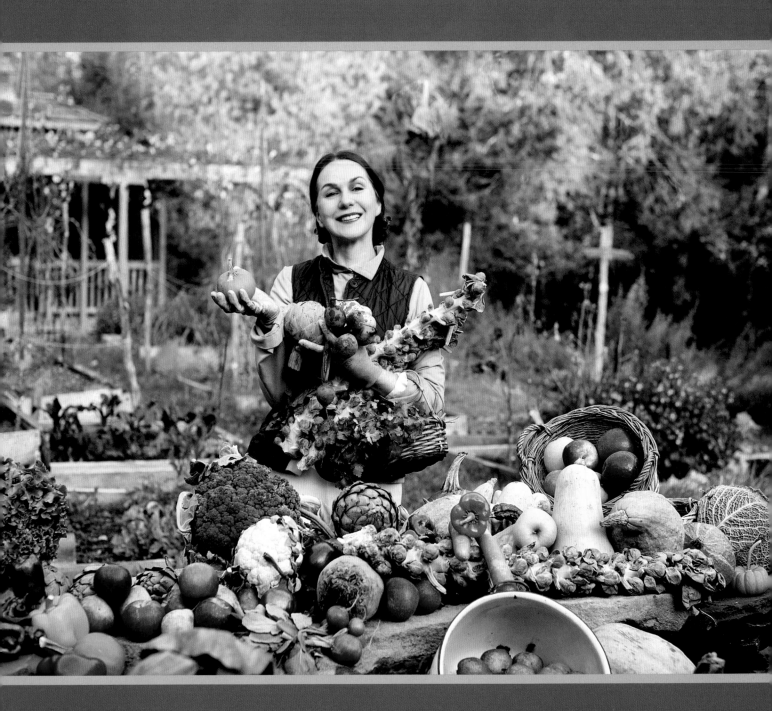

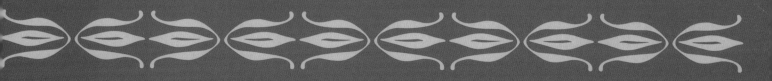

Vegetables

Although all of the dishes in this book can be considered vegetables because they are all plant based, this chapter focuses on vegetables that are prepared separately from grains, beans, and pulses and are not prepared in a soup, dessert, or drink. Many of the dishes in this chapter can be served alone as side dishes or mixed with noodles, rice, or other grains.

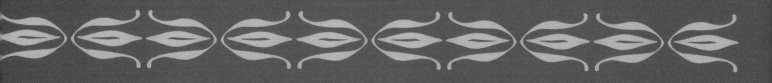

⋙ Simple Steamed Veggies ⋘

Using a steamer is a must for this recipe. It is good to invest in a stainless-steel
double steamer, so you can put vegetables that need more cooking time
(like potatoes, carrots, or winter squash) in the bottom basket and vegetables
that need less cooking time (like kale, collards,
and mustard greens) in the top.

Your favorite vegetables, washed and cut into pieces

Fill the bottom of a steamer pot with water and bring to a boil over high heat. Place the vegetables in the steamer basket, cover the pot with a tight-fitting lid, and steam until the vegetables are bright in color and tender.

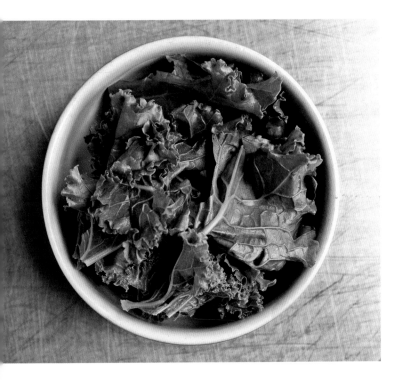
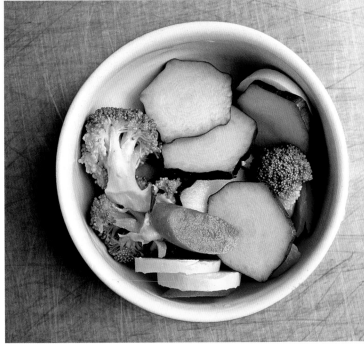

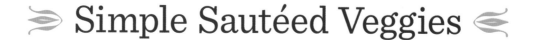

Simple Sautéed Veggies

The amount of time you sauté the vegetables will depend on what type of vegetables you are cooking. Root vegetables will take longer than green and most aboveground vegetables.

Olive oil
Your favorite vegetable(s), washed and cut into slices or pieces
Salt and freshly ground black pepper to taste

In a frying pan large enough to hold all the vegetables, heat enough oil to over the bottom of the pan over medium heat and add the vegetables. Cook, stirring often, for 1 minute, then reduce the heat to low and cover the pan with a tight-fitting lid. Cook until the vegetables reach the desired consistency. Add salt and pepper to taste.

⇒ Sautéed Collards ⇐
with Herbs

Collard greens are a hearty plant and have a long growing season;
the same plant can even overwinter, providing an abundance nearly all year round.

½ cup olive oil

6 collard greens leaves, chopped into
   very small pieces

2 cloves garlic, finely chopped

1 teaspoon fresh rosemary, fresh
   oregano, and/or fresh thyme, finely
   chopped

Salt and freshly ground black pepper
   to taste

In a large frying pan, heat the olive oil over medium heat. Add the greens, garlic, rosemary, oregano, and thyme and sauté for 1 minute, stirring continuously. Reduce the heat to low, cover the pan with a tight-fitting lid, and cook for 1 to 3 minutes longer, until the greens are the desired consistency. Add salt and pepper to taste.

SERVES 4 TO 6

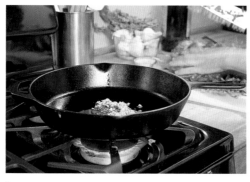

1.

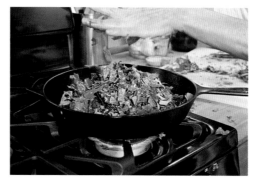

2.

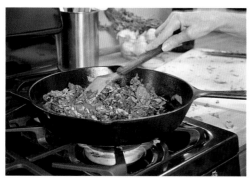

3.

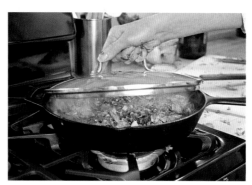

4.

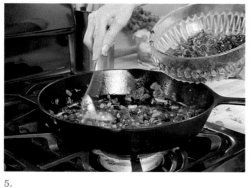

5.

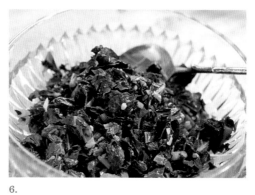

6.

Sautéed Kale and Potatoes

Quick and tasty, this recipe is made from staples from my Woodstock garden.

½ cup olive oil

2 cloves garlic, chopped

1 teaspoon dried oregano

6 leaves kale, chopped into small
    pieces

1 cooked potato, peeled or unpeeled
    and diced small

Salt and freshly ground black pepper
    to taste

In a large frying pan, heat the olive oil over medium heat. Add the garlic and oregano and sauté for 1 minute. Add the kale and potatoes, reduce the heat to low, cover the pan with a tight-fitting lid, and cook for 3 to 5 more minutes, until the kale and potatoes are tender. Season with salt and pepper to taste.

SERVES 4 TO 6

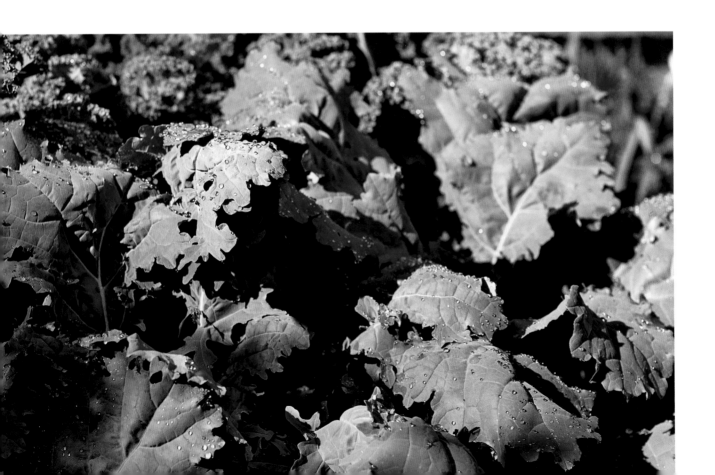

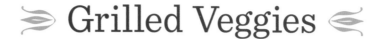 Grilled Veggies

This basic recipe calls for only olive oil and salt, but these veggies
can be seasoned with any spices or herbs you like.

1 medium zucchini, cut in ¼-inch rounds

1 large yellow squash, cut in ¼-inch
rounds

2 medium potatoes, peeled or unpeeled
and cut into thin rounds or long
strips

1 red, green, or yellow bell pepper, cut
into slices

3 tablespoons olive oil

1 tablespoon salt

In a large bowl, place the zucchini, squash, potatoes, bell pepper, olive oil, and salt and toss to mix well. Arrange the vegetables on a grill and cook for about 3 minutes, until grill marks appear on the bottom side of the squash, then turn and grill for another 3 minutes. Alternatively, broil the vegetables in an oven for about the same amount of time, turning once.

SERVES 4 TO 6

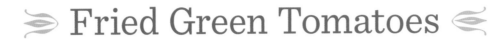

Fried Green Tomatoes

In the summertime, when I was growing up in Washington, D.C., my grandmother would buy green tomatoes from a cart on the street and fry them up. This is close to the recipe that I remember, with the exception of the corn chips, which is my personal addition.

½ cup olive oil

½ red onion, chopped

4 cloves garlic, chopped

4 medium green tomatoes (1¼ to 1½ pounds), sliced

¼ teaspoon red pepper flakes

½ teaspoon ground cumin

½ teaspoon paprika

½ teaspoon celery seeds

½ teaspoon dried oregano

¼ cup water

1 cup corn chips

Salt to taste

In a large frying pan, heat the olive oil over medium-high heat. Add the onion and garlic and sauté for 5 to 10 minutes, until the onions are translucent. Add the tomatoes, red pepper flakes, cumin, paprika, celery seeds, and oregano and sauté for about 3 minutes, turning at least once, until well mixed. Add the water, reduce the heat to medium-low, and cook, covered, for 10 minutes, or until the tomatoes are soft, adding more water if needed to yield a sauce-like consistency. Add the corn chips and salt to taste, stir, and cook for another minute.

SERVES 4 TO 6

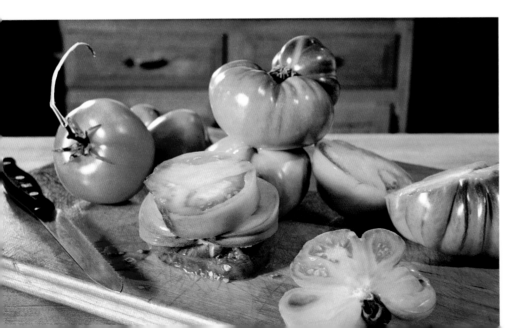

⇒ Jambalaya ⇐

This is my Cajun-Mexican version of this "jumbled-up" jambalaya.

¼ cup olive oil

3 cloves garlic, finely chopped

1 tablespoon dried oregano

1 teaspoon ground cumin

1 teaspoon ground coriander

1 teaspoon Cajun spice seasoning

3 medium green tomatoes (about
   1 pound), sliced

1 ripe red tomato, sliced

1 green or red bell pepper, sliced

½ cup water

One 15-ounce can black-eyed peas, with
   liquid

½ cup fresh or frozen corn kernels

½ teaspoon salt, plus more to taste

1 cup cooked white rice

4 fresh or frozen corn tortillas

Vegan sour cream to taste

Commercially prepared tomato salsa
   to taste

In a large frying pan, heat the olive oil over medium heat. Add the garlic, oregano, cumin, coriander, and Cajun spices and sauté for 1 minute. Add the green and red tomatoes and bell pepper, reduce the heat to medium-low, and cook, covered with a tight-fitting lid, for about 10 minutes, or until the vegetables are soft. Reduce the heat to low. Add the water, black-eyed peas, corn, and salt and simmer, covered, for 5 minutes, until the flavors are well blended. Add the rice and mix well. Place the tortillas over the mixture, replace the lid, turn off the heat, and allow the mixture to sit for about 5 minutes to soften the tortillas. Spoon the mixture into individual bowls, keeping the tortillas on top. Sprinkle with salt to taste, and top with a dollop of sour cream and salsa to taste.

SERVES 4 TO 6

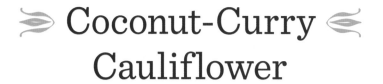 Coconut-Curry Cauliflower

I've traveled several times to Southeast Asia and miss the delicate
flavors of the cuisine. I have tried to replicate them here.

1 head cauliflower, broken into florets

3 tablespoons vegetable oil

1 tablespoon mustard seeds

One 2-inch piece fresh ginger, peeled
   and coarsely chopped

½ teaspoon red pepper flakes

1 cup water

1 medium potato, peeled and diced into
   small pieces

1 teaspoon turmeric powder

1 teaspoon ground cumin

1 teaspoon ground coriander

1 teaspoon curry powder

1 teaspoon sugar

1 teaspoon salt

One 10- to 15-ounce can coconut milk

12 ounces firm or extra-firm tofu, cut
   into ½-inch cubes

1 tomato, cut into small pieces

½ cup chopped fresh cilantro

Cooked rice, for serving

In a steamer basket set over boiling water, place the cauliflower and steam for 5 to 6 minutes,
until tender but still firm; set aside.

In a small frying pan, heat the vegetable oil over medium heat. Add the mustard seeds, cover,
and sauté for about 1 minute, until the seeds pop, taking care not to let them burn. Add the ginger
and red pepper flakes and cook for 3 minutes. Add the water, potato, turmeric, cumin, coriander,
curry powder, sugar, and salt. Reduce the heat to medium-low and cook for 10 to 15 minutes,
until the potatoes are soft. Add the coconut milk, then remove from the heat and allow to cool for
10 minutes.

Transfer the sautéed ingredients to the bowl of a food processor or blender and blend until
creamy. Transfer the blended ingredients back to the frying pan, add the cauliflower, tofu, coconut milk, tomato, and cilantro, and stir well. Serve over rice.

SERVES 4 TO 6

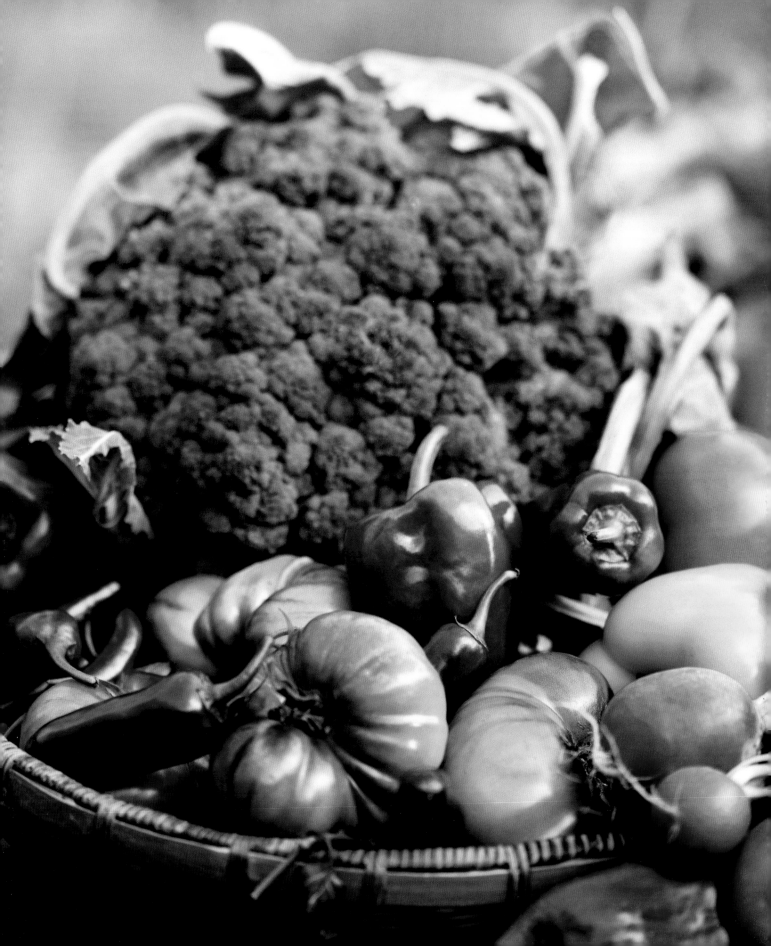

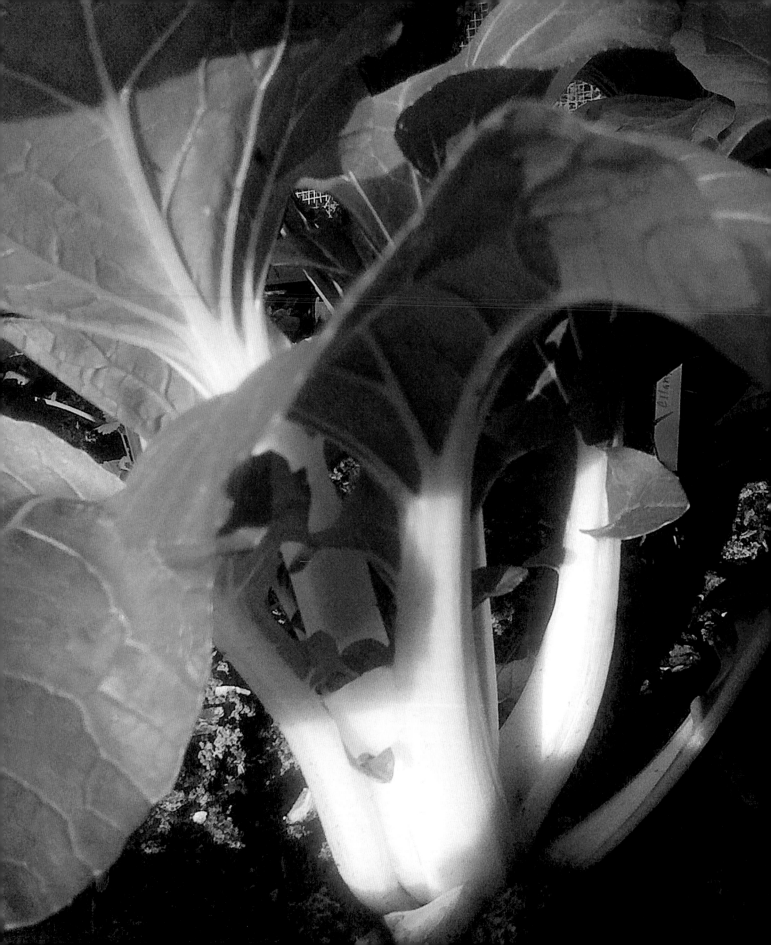

⤜ Stir-Fried Vegetables, ⤛ Chinese Style

This dish works well with any vegetables. I've chosen ones that traditionally
appear in chop suey, and I've added pineapple for some sweetness.

6 dried shiitake mushrooms

½ cup safflower oil, peanut oil, or
   sesame oil

One ½-inch piece fresh ginger, peeled
   and finely chopped

1 stalk celery, cut on an angle into thin
   slices

1 carrot, peeled and cut on an angle into
   thin slices

1 stalk bok choy, cut on an angle

1 cup broccoli florets

1 green or red bell pepper, sliced into
   thin strips

10 pea pods, whole

One 4-ounce can sliced water chestnuts

One 4-ounce can sliced bamboo shoots

1 tablespoon organic non-GMO
   cornstarch

1 cup cold water

1 tablespoon soy sauce, tamari, or
   Braggs Liquid Aminos

1 teaspoon Chinese five-spice powder

¼ teaspoon cayenne pepper

One 8-ounce can pineapple chunks with
   unsweetened juice

Cooked rice or noodles, for serving

In a small bowl, place the mushrooms and add boiling water to cover, and let stand for 5 to
10 minutes to rehydrate. Drain, then slice the mushrooms into strips and set aside.

In a large frying pan or wok, heat the safflower oil over medium-high heat. Add the ginger and
fry for 1 minute, stirring continuously. Add the mushrooms, celery, carrot, bok choy, broccoli, and
bell pepper and cook for another 2 minutes. Add the pea pods, water chestnuts, and bamboo
shoots and turn off the heat.

Place the cornstarch in a cup or medium bowl. Add the water and stir until smooth and
creamy. Add the soy sauce, five-spice powder, cayenne, and pineapple and mix well.

Add the mixture to the frying pan and stir. Return to medium heat and cook, uncovered, for
3 to 5 minutes, until well mixed and well heated. Serve over rice or noodles.

SERVES 4 TO 6

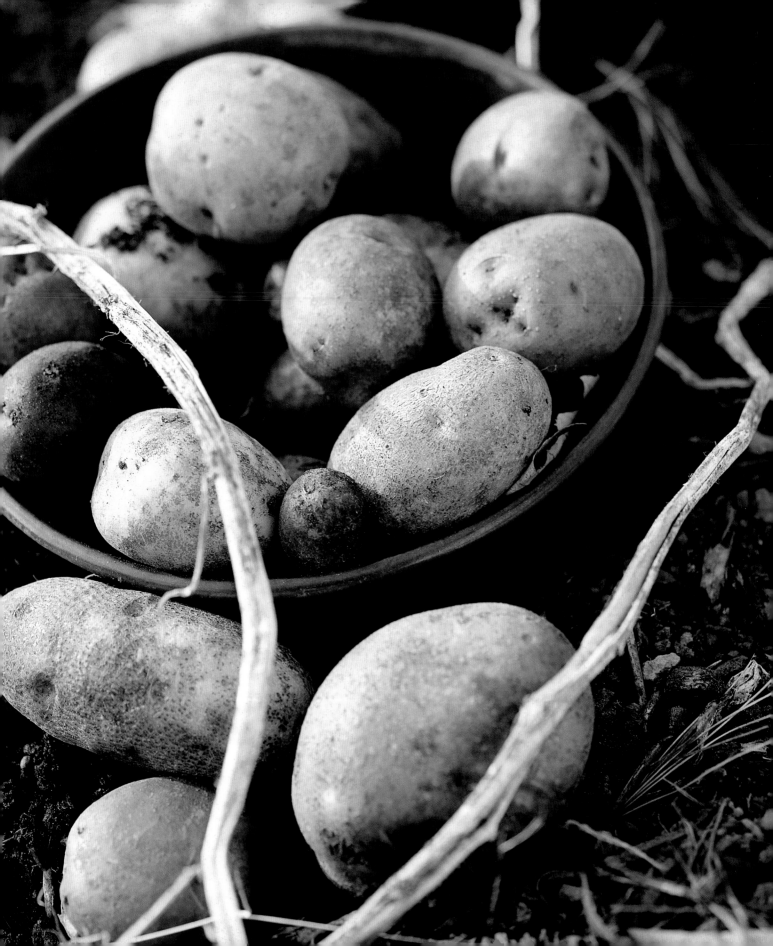

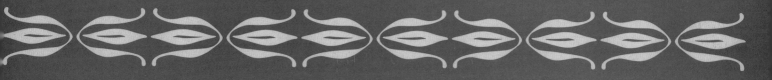

Potatoes

The potato is a versatile, starchy root vegetable containing complex carbohydrates, vitamin C, and even protein, and it is low in calories. Because of its bland taste, it offers itself as a primed canvas ready to manifest the creativity of any chef. Because I am Irish, potatoes deserve their own chapter in my book.

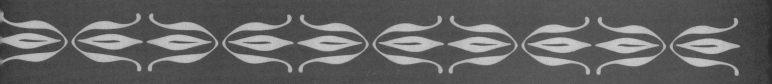

⮁ Simple Steamed Potatoes ⮀

5 to 6 potatoes, skins scrubbed, cut into medium or small pieces

In a steamer basket set over boiling water, place the potatoes and steam for about 15 minutes, until tender. Serve plain or with any of the toppings suggested for Baked Potatoes (page 226).

SERVES 4 TO 6

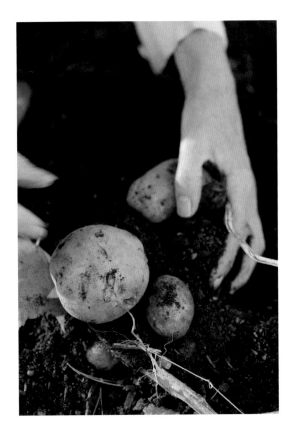 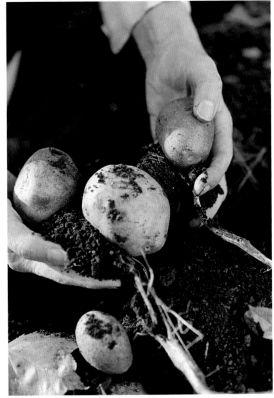

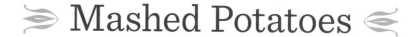

Mashed Potatoes

This is the ultimate comfort food, and comfort here means not only for the diner but also for the dairy cows whose milk and cream we have not stolen. And here's a tip: when you drain the boiled potatoes, reserve the cooking water for use as soup stock.

6 potatoes (2 to 3 pounds), scrubbed clean or peeled and cut into small pieces
¼ cup olive oil
Salt and freshly ground black pepper to taste

½ to ¾ cup soy milk or almond milk, depending on the desired consistency

In a large saucepan, place the potatoes and just enough water to cover, and bring to a boil and cook for about 20 minutes, until you can stick a fork through a potato easily. Drain the potatoes. Return them to the saucepan and add the olive oil and salt and pepper to taste, then gradually add the soy milk as you mash with a potato masher until creamy and smooth, or use an electric hand mixer. Add more soy milk as needed to obtain the desired consistency.

VARIATION

Substitute 2 parsnips for 2 of the potatoes.

SERVES 4 TO 6

⇝ Parsley, Sage, Rosemary, ⇜ and Thyme Mashed Potatoes

This is a perfect dish to bring to a potluck at Scarborough Fair.

6 potatoes (2 to 3 pounds), scrubbed clean or peeled and cut into small pieces

4 tablespoons olive oil, divided

1 tablespoon dried sage

1 tablespoon dried rosemary

1 tablespoon dried thyme

1 cup soy milk or almond milk

2 tablespoons finely chopped fresh parsley

Salt and freshly ground black pepper to taste

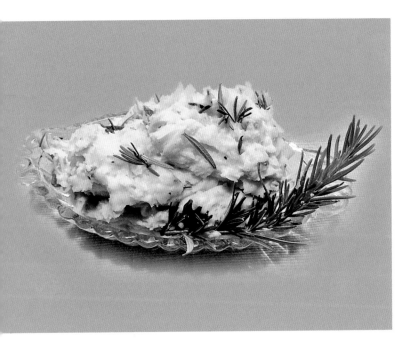

In a large saucepan, place the potatoes and just enough water to cover, then bring to a boil and cook for about 20 minutes, until you can stick a fork through a potato easily. Remove from the heat, cover the pot, and set aside.

In a small frying pan, heat 1 tablespoon of the olive oil. Add the sage, rosemary, and thyme and sauté for 1 to 2 minutes, taking care not to let the herbs burn.

Drain the potatoes, return them to the saucepan, add the soy milk and remaining 3 tablespoons olive oil, and mash with a potato masher until creamy and smooth, or use an electric hand mixer. Stir in the sautéed herbs, parsley, and salt and pepper to taste.

SERVES 4 TO 6

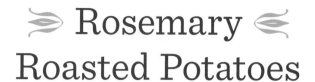

Rosemary Roasted Potatoes

Warning: While these potatoes are roasting, your entire home will be filled with an herby, heavenly aroma.

6 potatoes (2 to 3 pounds), unpeeled and cut into bite-size pieces

2 tablespoons olive oil

2 tablespoons dried rosemary

Salt and freshly ground black pepper to taste

In a 9 x 13-inch glass baking dish, place the potatoes, pour the olive oil over the potatoes, sprinkle with rosemary and salt and pepper to taste, and let sit while you preheat the oven to 375°F. When the oven is ready, bake for about 30 minutes, or until browned and tender.

SERVES 4 TO 6

⋙ Baked Potatoes ⋘

The easiest way to prepare potatoes, and the infinite range of topping
alternatives makes them appropriate for any meal. I particularly like
to lavish my potato with Turmeric-Tahini Dressing (page 159).

6 large russet potatoes, skins scrubbed

Preheat the oven to 350°F. Oil a 9 x 9-inch baking pan.

Prick potatoes several times with a fork. In the prepared pan, place potatoes and bake for
45 minutes. Remove from the oven, slice open, and add toppings of your choice.

SERVES 6

⋙ Baked Potato Toppings ⋘

Salt and freshly ground black pepper

Vegan margarine, salt, and freshly
ground black pepper

Vegan margarine and stone-ground
mustard

Vegan margarine, salt, freshly ground
black pepper, and chopped fresh
parsley

Olive oil, salt, and freshly ground black
pepper

Olive oil, salt, freshly ground black
pepper, and dried tarragon

Olive oil, salt, freshly ground black
pepper, and dried oregano

Olive oil, salt, freshly ground black
pepper, and grated vegan cheese

Olive oil, salt, red pepper flakes, and
tofu sour cream

Toasted sesame oil and soy sauce,
tamari, or Braggs Liquid Aminos

Cubes of Marinated Tofu (page 204)

Flaxseed oil, salt, and freshly ground
black pepper

Pesto (page 98)

Any dressing of your choice (see
pages 152–160)

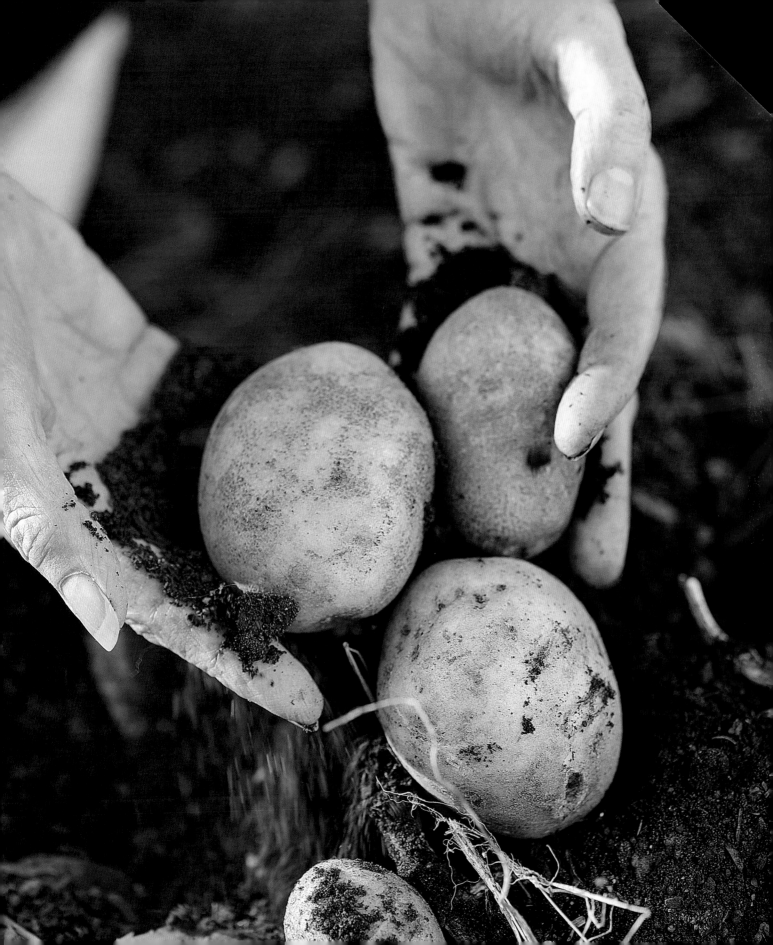

⇝ Shepherd's Pie ⇜

Here is a vegan version of the classic cuisine of my Irish ancestors.

2 tablespoons olive oil

1 large onion, finely chopped

2 cloves garlic, finely chopped

1 green bell pepper, chopped

1 teaspoon dried oregano

1 teaspoon dried rosemary

½ cup peas

½ cup green beans, cut into ½-inch
  pieces

1 tablespoon chopped fresh parsley

One 12-ounce package commercially
  prepared vegan ground beef

One 12-ounce jar commercially
  prepared tomato sauce, or
  homemade Tomato Sauce (from
  Pasta with Tomato Sauce, page 103)

Mashed Potatoes (page 223), prepared

½ cup shredded vegan Cheddar cheese

Preheat the oven to 400°F.

In a large cast-iron frying pan, heat the olive oil over medium-high heat. Add the onion, garlic, bell pepper, oregano, and rosemary and sauté for 2 minutes. Stir in the peas, green beans, parsley, vegan ground beef, and tomato sauce and mix well. Remove from the heat and top with the mashed potatoes, sprinkle the cheese on top, and bake for about 20 minutes, until the cheese melts and the potatoes are slightly browned.

SERVES 6 TO 8

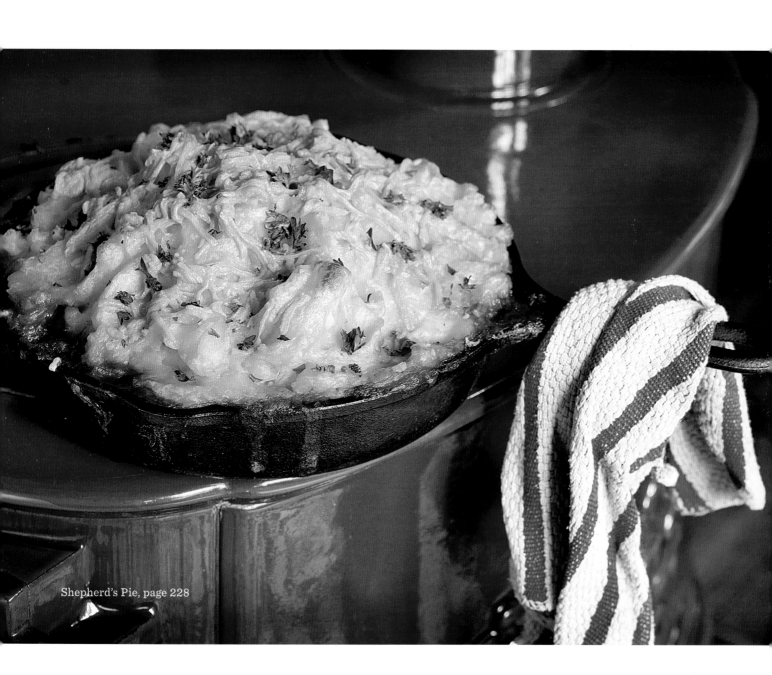

Shepherd's Pie, page 228

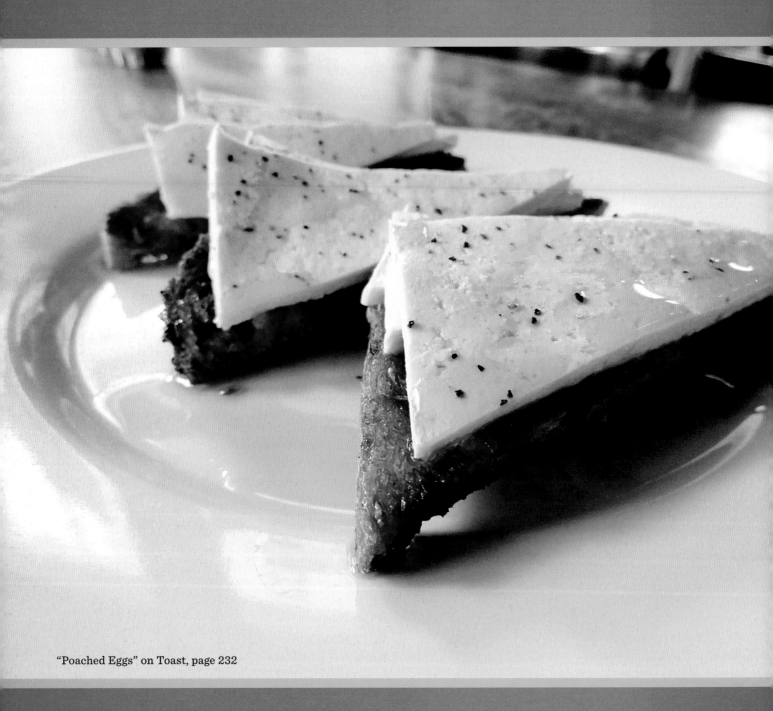

"Poached Eggs" on Toast, page 232

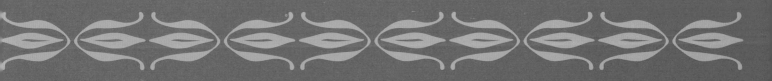

Toasts

My favorite meal is tea and toast. At Jivamuktea Café
we serve a large variety of our own house blends of organic teas, which all go well with toast for breakfast or
as a snack any time of the day. Following are several
ideas.

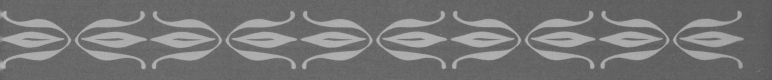

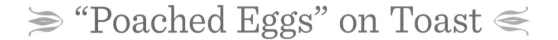

"Poached Eggs" on Toast

The combination of tofu and flaxseed oil surprisingly tastes like a poached egg.

2 slices bread
1 to 2 tablespoons flaxseed oil
1 tablespoon vegan margarine

Two ¼-inch slices firm tofu
Salt and freshly ground black pepper
to taste

Toast the bread in a toaster. Spread flaxseed oil lavishly on the toast, then "butter" the toast lightly with margarine. Place 1 slice of tofu on each slice of toast, drizzle a few drops of flaxseed oil over the tofu, and sprinkle with salt and pepper to taste.

SERVES 1

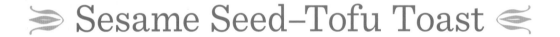

Sesame Seed–Tofu Toast

This may be the first original recipe I ever came up with. I used to eat this nearly every day during college, once I discovered the delights of tofu and a toaster oven.

2 slices bread
2 tablespoons vegan mayonnaise

2 tablespoons sesame seeds
Two ¼-inch slices cold firm tofu

Spread mayonnaise on each slice of bread, sprinkle with the sesame seeds, then place the bread under the broiler of a toaster oven and cook until the bread crusts are toasted and the sesame seeds begin to pop. Remove from the oven and lay the tofu slices on top.

SERVES 1

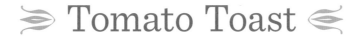

Tomato Toast

This speaks for itself.

2 slices bread

2 tablespoons olive oil, plus more as
needed

4 large slices tomato, red or green

Salt and freshly ground black pepper to
taste

4 leaves arugula or fresh basil

Toast the bread in a toaster. Drizzle the olive oil over the toast. Lay the tomato slices on the toast, sprinkle with salt and pepper to taste, top with the basil, and drizzle more oil on top.

SERVES 1

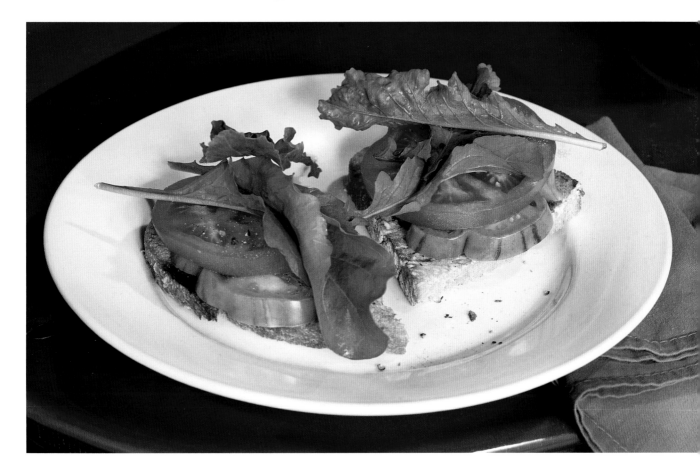

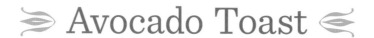

Avocado Toast

Enjoy this on its own or simply add a slice of tomato to
make a "TAVO," which is a favorite at Jivamuktea Café.

2 slices bread

1 tablespoon vegan margarine

½ avocado, thinly sliced

1 tablespoon flaxseed oil

Salt and freshly ground black pepper to
taste

Toast the bread in a toaster. "Butter" the toast lightly with the margarine, lay the avocado slices
on the toast, drizzle a few drops of flaxseed oil over the avocado, and sprinkle with salt and pepper to taste.

SERVES 1

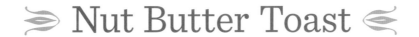 Nut Butter Toast

When I was eight years old, my grandmother spontaneously
made an open-faced peanut butter sandwich and topped it with
lettuce. She was as excited about this discovery as when
she first saw color TV. Me too.

2 slices bread
2 tablespoons almond butter or peanut butter
2 leaves any kind of lettuce or arugula

Toast the bread in a toaster. Spread the toast with the almond butter and lay the lettuce leaves on top.

SERVES 1

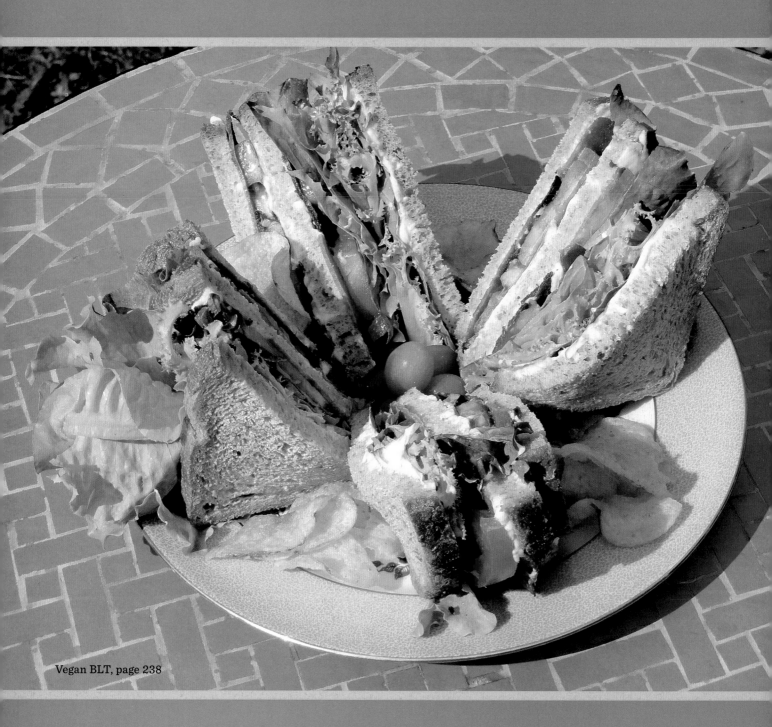

Vegan BLT, page 238

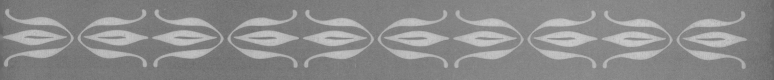

Sandwiches

Traditionally, a sandwich is defined as two or more slices of bread with one or more fillings in between. I extend that definition to include burritos and quesadillas. Sandwiches are basic fare at any café, and at Jivamuktea Café we offer many delectable concoctions.

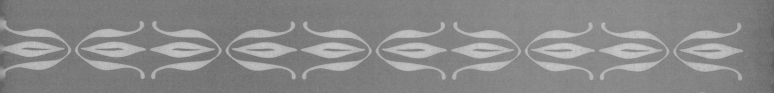

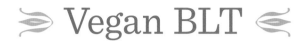 Vegan BLT

One of my bacon-loving friends says he can't tell the difference between this and a "real" BLT. Try enjoying this sandwich along with some organic potato chips!

1 tablespoon olive oil

4 thin slices commercially prepared vegan bacon

3 slices bread

2 tablespoons vegan mayonnaise

1 large tomato, sliced

2 leaves any kind of lettuce

In a medium frying pan, heat the olive oil over medium-high heat. Add the bacon and sauté until crisp.

Toast the bread and liberally spread each slice with the mayonnaise. Lay 2 slices of bacon on 1 slice of toast. Top with a few slices of tomato and a lettuce leaf. Cover with another slice of toast, the remaining 2 slices of bacon, the remaining slices of tomato, the remaining lettuce leaf, and the third slice of toast, mayonnaise side down, creating a triple-decker sandwich. Cut into quarters.

SERVES 1

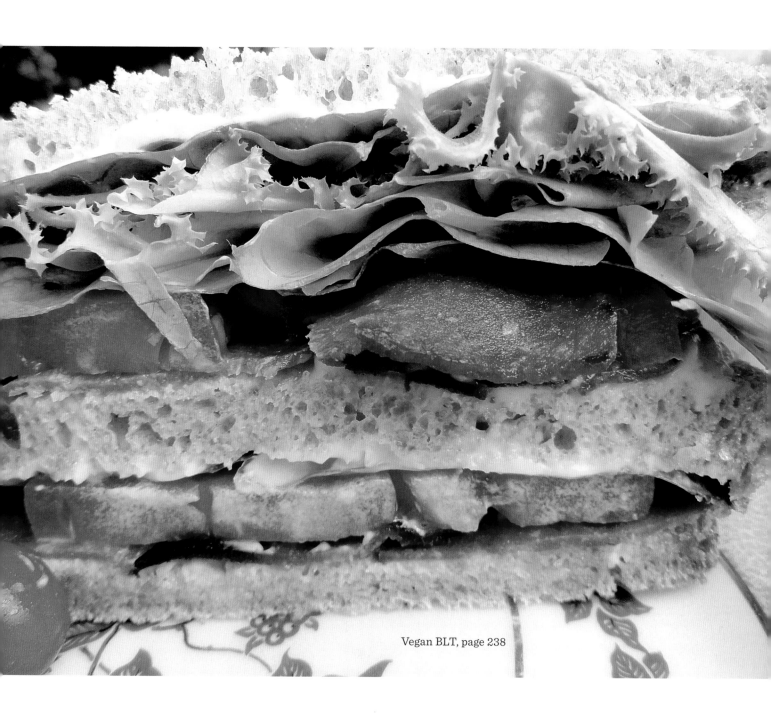

Vegan BLT, page 238

⇒ Grilled Portabella ⇐ Mushroom Panini

Jivamuktea Café in New York City is not zoned for a gas stove and exhaust system, so we cleverly found a way to manage through induction burners and a panini grill. All of our hot sandwiches are made on this grill, much to the delight of our diners.

1 tablespoon Chimichurri Sauce
  (page 160)
2 slices bread
One 2-inch portabella mushroom cap,
  grilled, or ¼ cup sliced and sautéed
  mushrooms (any kind)

2 tablespoons sautéed chopped onions
1 teaspoon nutritional yeast flakes
Olive oil

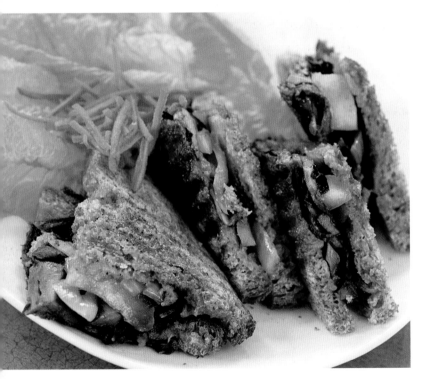

Drizzle the chimichurri sauce on both slices of bread. Cut the mushroom cap to fit on 1 slice of the bread, or place the sautéed mushrooms on 1 slice of the bread. Layer the onions over the mushrooms. Sprinkle the nutritional yeast on the onions and top with the other slice of bread.

Brush a panini grill with olive oil. Place the sandwich on the grill and brush it with oil. Close the grill and cook for about 2 minutes, or until grill marks appear. (Or, in a small frying pan, heat at least 2 tablespoons of olive oil over medium heat. Brush the sandwich with olive oil and place it in the frying pan. Allow it to cook for 2 minutes on one side, then flip and cook for 2 minutes on the other side.)

SERVES 1

⇒ Grilled Veggie Panini ⇐

2 tablespoons Hummus (page 165)

2 slices bread

⅓ cup Simple Steamed Veggies
  (page 208)—your choice (zucchini,
  red bell pepper, eggplant, and
  tomato work well)

1 teaspoon spirulina powder

1 tablespoon Balsamic Vinaigrette
  (page 156)

Olive oil

Spread the hummus on 1 slice of bread. Layer the vegetables over the hummus and sprinkle with the spirulina powder. Drizzle the balsamic vinaigrette on the other slice of bread and lay it on top.

Brush a panini grill with olive oil. Place the sandwich on the grill and brush it with oil. Close the grill and cook for about 2 minutes, or until grill marks appear. (Or, in a small frying pan, heat at least 2 tablespoons of olive oil over medium heat. Brush the sandwich with olive oil and place it in the frying pan. Allow it to cook for 2 minutes on one side, then flip and cook for 2 minutes on the other side.)

SERVES 1

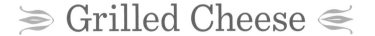 Grilled Cheese

One of the things that many new vegans miss most is grilled cheese,
but not once they taste this sandwich.

2 slices bread

1 tablespoon vegan margarine

¼ cup grated commercially prepared
vegan cheese

1 teaspoon nutritional yeast

Olive oil

"Butter" both slices of bread with the margarine. Spread the grated cheese evenly on 1 slice, and sprinkle the nutritional yeast over the cheese. Place the other slice of bread on top.

Brush a panini grill with olive oil. Place the sandwich on the grill and brush it with oil. Close the grill and cook for about 2 minutes, or until grill marks appear. (Or, in a small frying pan, heat at least 2 tablespoons of olive oil over medium heat. Brush the sandwich with olive oil and place it in the frying pan. Allow it to cook for 2 minutes on one side, then flip and cook for 2 minutes on the other side.)

SERVES 1

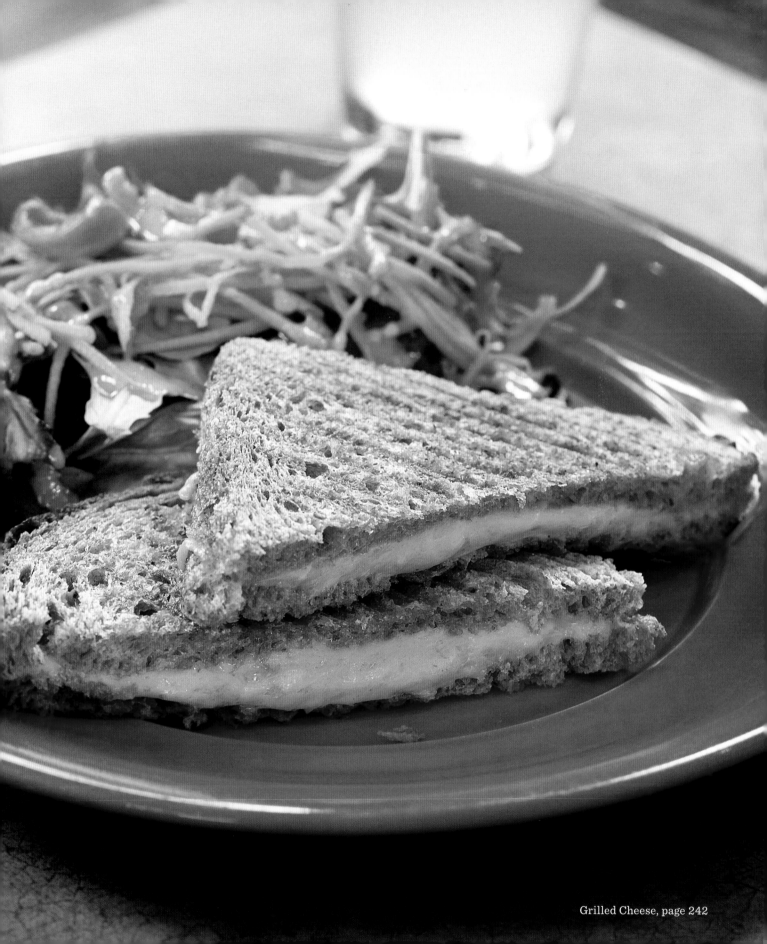

Grilled Cheese, page 242

⋙ Vegan Bacon Quesadilla ⋘

In Jivamuktea Café, we call this Vegan Bacon QuesaDaiya after
the Daiya brand of vegan cheese alternative cleverly made from green peas.
We were the first restaurant in New York to try out this brand commercially.

3 slices commercially prepared vegan
   bacon
1 whole-wheat tortilla
Freshly ground black pepper or red
   pepper flakes to taste

1 teaspoon diced onion (optional)
½ tomato, diced
¼ cup grated commercially prepared
   vegan cheese
Olive oil

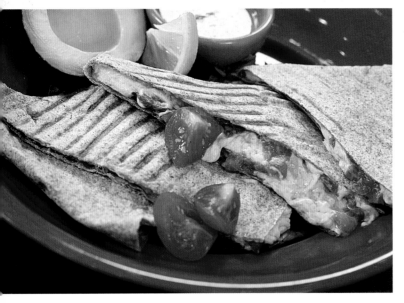

Grill or pan-fry the bacon. Lay the tortilla flat
and sprinkle it with pepper to taste. Layer the
bacon, onion, tomato, and cheese on one side,
then fold the tortilla in half.

Brush a panini grill with olive oil. Place the
tortilla on the grill and brush with oil. Close
the grill and cook for about 2 minutes, or until
grill marks appear. (Or, in a small frying pan,
heat at least 2 tablespoons of olive oil over medium heat. Brush the tortilla with olive oil and
place it in the frying pan. Allow it to cook for
2 minutes on one side, then flip and cook for
2 minutes on the other side.)

SERVES 1

⇒ Grilled Nut Butter ⇐ and Jelly

This is great for kids of all ages.

2 slices bread

1 tablespoon vegan margarine

2 tablespoons almond butter, peanut butter, or cashew butter

1 tablespoon raspberry jam (or any other jam of your choice)

Olive oil

"Butter" both slices of bread with the margarine. Spread the nut butter evenly on 1 slice of bread, then spread the jam on top of the nut butter. Place the other slice of bread on top.

Brush a panini grill with olive oil. Place the sandwich on the grill and brush it with oil. Close the grill and cook for about 2 minutes, or until grill marks appear. (Or, in a small frying pan, heat at least 2 tablespoons of olive oil over medium heat. Brush the sandwich with olive oil and place it in the frying pan. Allow it to cook for 2 minutes on one side, then flip and cook for 2 minutes on the other side.)

SERVES 1

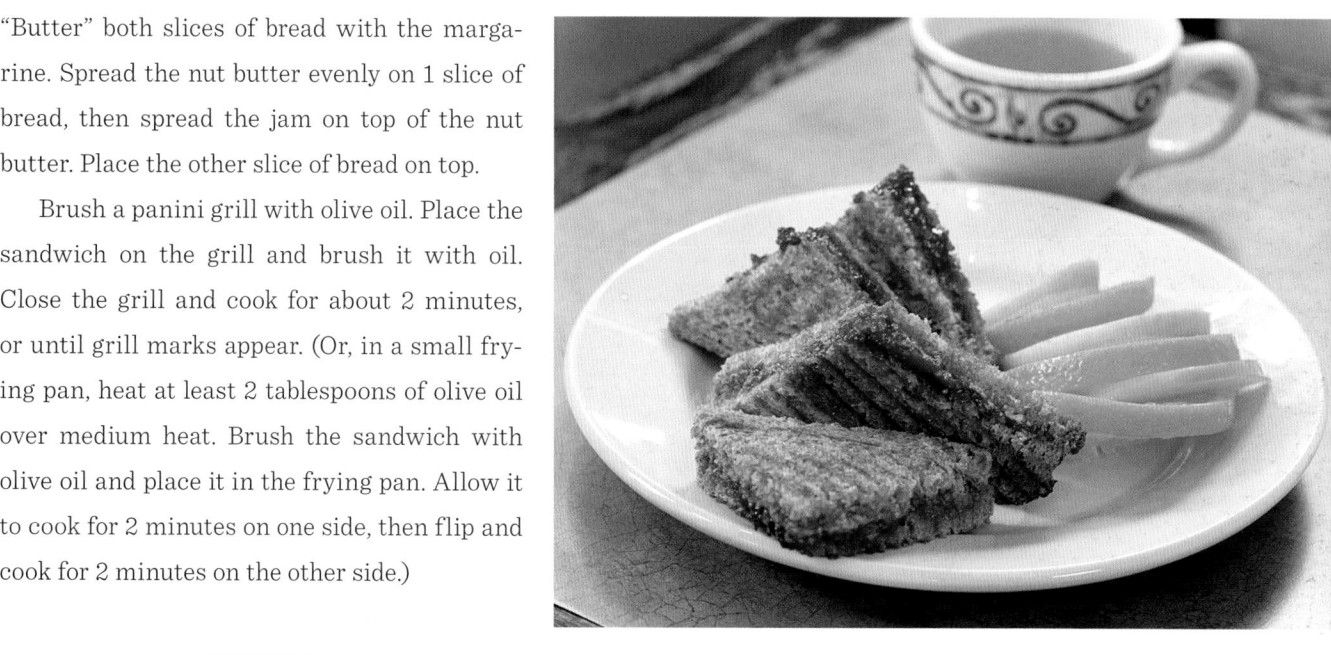

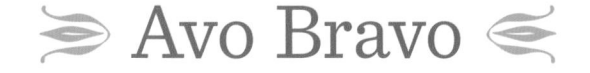 Avo Bravo

This is like a salad in a sandwich.

2 tablespoons Turmeric-Tahini Dressing (page 159)

2 slices bread, toasted, if desired

½ avocado, thinly sliced

½ Granny Smith apple, cored and thinly sliced

½ cup shredded lettuce (preferably romaine)

1 tablespoon grated peeled carrot

Spread the dressing on both slices of bread. Lay the avocado on 1 slice, then top with the apples and then the lettuce. Sprinkle with grated carrot, then place the other slice of bread on top and cut diagonally in half.

SERVES 1

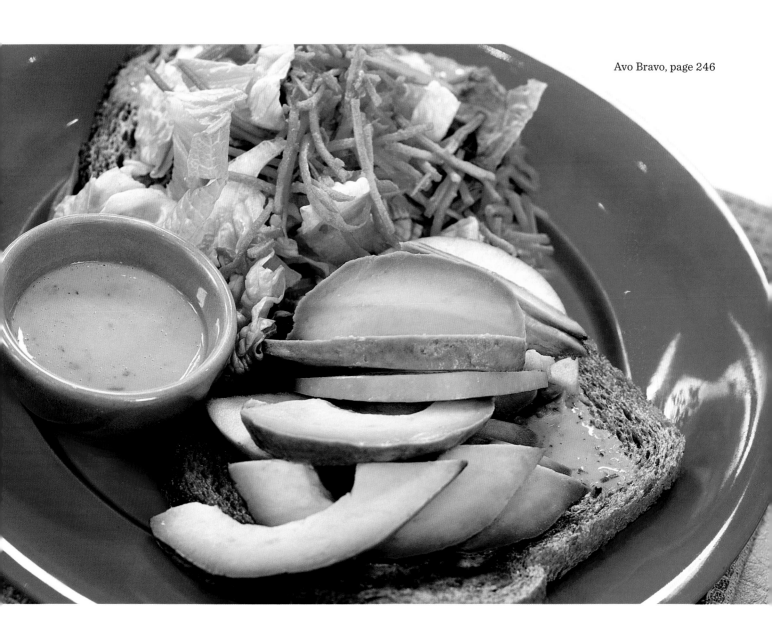

Avo Bravo, page 246

≥ Insteada-Tuna ≤ Salad Sandwich

You won't believe that the main ingredient of the "tuna" is uncooked tempeh—gone fish-ing.

2 slices bread

2 tablespoons (¼ stick) vegan margarine

¼ cup Insteada-Tuna Salad (page 147)

1 leaf romaine lettuce, or any other kind

"Butter" both slices of bread with the margarine. Spread the tuna salad on 1 slice. Lay the lettuce on top of the tuna salad and place the other slice of bread on top. Cut diagonally in half.

SERVES 1

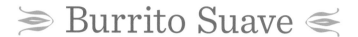 Burrito Suave

I developed this and the other burritos with a former manager at Jivamuktea Café,
David Armstrong, who is from the American Southwest and a master of Tex-Mex cuisine.

One 12-inch whole-wheat tortilla

½ cup cooked brown rice

⅓ cup Black Beans (see page 190)

⅓ cup Smoky Pinto Beans (see
   page 191)

¼ cup chopped tomatoes

1 tablespoon diced onions

¼ avocado, cut into strips

2 leaves romaine lettuce, shredded

1 tablespoon Chimichurri Sauce (see
   page 160)

Olive oil

Lay the tortilla flat and spread the rice across the middle. Spread the black beans and pinto beans over the rice. Layer the tomatoes, onions, avocado, and lettuce on top of the rice and beans and drizzle with the sauce. Fold the edge of the tortilla closest to you toward the middle of the mixture, then repeat with the opposite edge. Then, starting with the right side, begin to fold the tortilla up slowly, ensuring that the folded sides remain intact. Continue until the burrito is completely enclosed.

Brush a panini press with olive oil and press the burrito for 30 seconds to seal. (Or, in a small frying pan, heat about 1 tablespoon of olive oil over medium heat and fry the burrito for 5 minutes, covered with a tight-fitting lid, until the edges of the burrito are sealed.)

SERVES 1

⋙ Burrito Verdura ⋘

One 12-inch whole-wheat tortilla

1 tablespoon commercially prepared
  vegan sour cream

½ cup Smoky Pinto Beans (see page 191)

½ cup Grilled Veggies (page 213) (using
  zucchini and yellow squash)

½ cup shredded commercially prepared
  vegan cheese

1 tablespoon Chimichurri Sauce (see
  page 160)

Olive oil

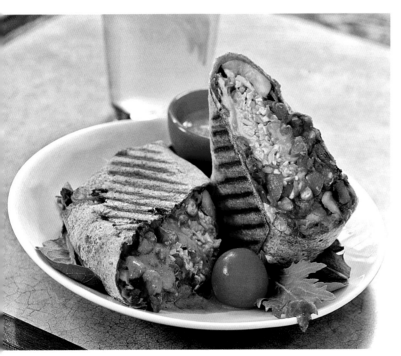

Lay the tortilla flat and spread the sour cream in the center. Layer the beans, vegetables, and cheese over the sour cream and drizzle with the sauce. Fold the edge of the tortilla closest to you toward the middle of the mixture, then repeat with the opposite edge. Then starting with the right side, begin to fold the tortilla up slowly, ensuring that the folded sides remain intact. Continue until the burrito is completely enclosed.

Brush a panini press with olive oil and press the burrito for 30 seconds to seal. (Or, in a small frying pan, heat about 1 tablespoon of olive oil over medium heat and fry the burrito for 5 minutes, covered with a tight-fitting lid, until the cheese melts and the edges of the burrito are sealed.)

SERVES 1

⇒ Burrito Diablo ⇐

One 12-inch whole-wheat tortilla

½ cup Rosemary Seitan (see page 197)

⅓ cup Black Beans (see page 190)

¼ cup chopped tomato

1 tablespoon diced onions

¼ avocado, cut into strips

2 leaves romaine lettuce, shredded

1 tablespoon Chimichurri Sauce (see
    page 160)

Olive oil

Lay the tortilla flat and lay the seitan in the center. Layer the beans, tomatoes, onions, avocado, and lettuce over the seitan, then drizzle with the sauce. Fold the edge of the tortilla closest to you toward the middle of the mixture, then repeat with the opposite edge. Then starting with the right side, begin to fold the tortilla up slowly, ensuring that the folded sides remain intact. Continue until the burrito is completely enclosed.

Brush a panini press with olive oil and press the burrito for 30 seconds to seal. (Or, in a small frying pan, heat about 1 tablespoon of olive oil over medium heat and fry the burrito for 5 minutes, covered with a tight-fitting lid, until the edges of the burrito are sealed.)

SERVES 1

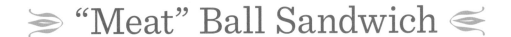 "Meat" Ball Sandwich

There was a place in Washington, DC, where my mother loved to eat that served a "Fill-more" meatball sandwich. I wish she were alive today to taste my vegan version.

One 8-inch sourdough bread roll

2 tablespoons (¼ stick) vegan margarine

¼ cup Tomato Sauce (from Pasta with Tomato Sauce, page 103)

5 "Meat" Balls (from Spaghetti and "Meat" Balls, page 104)

¼ cup shredded commercially prepared vegan mozzarella cheese, shredded

Slice the roll and "butter" both sides with the margarine. On one side of the roll spoon the tomato sauce, then place the "meat" balls in the sauce and sprinkle the cheese on top. Place both halves of the roll open-faced under a broiler for about 5 minutes, until the cheese melts. Remove from the broiler and close.

SERVES 1

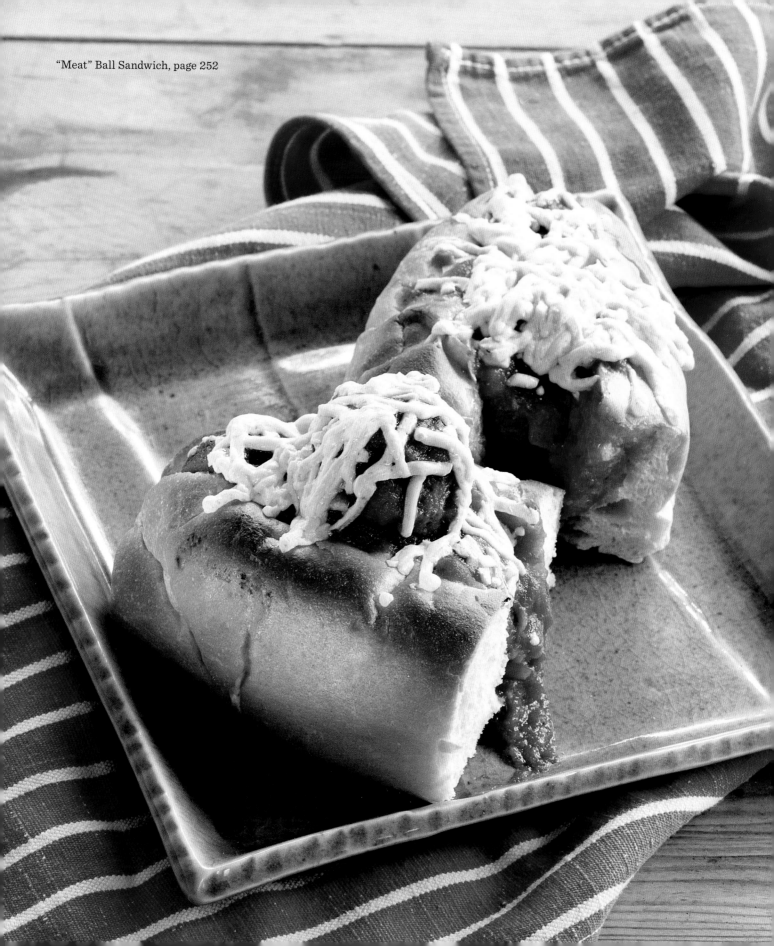

"Meat" Ball Sandwich, page 252

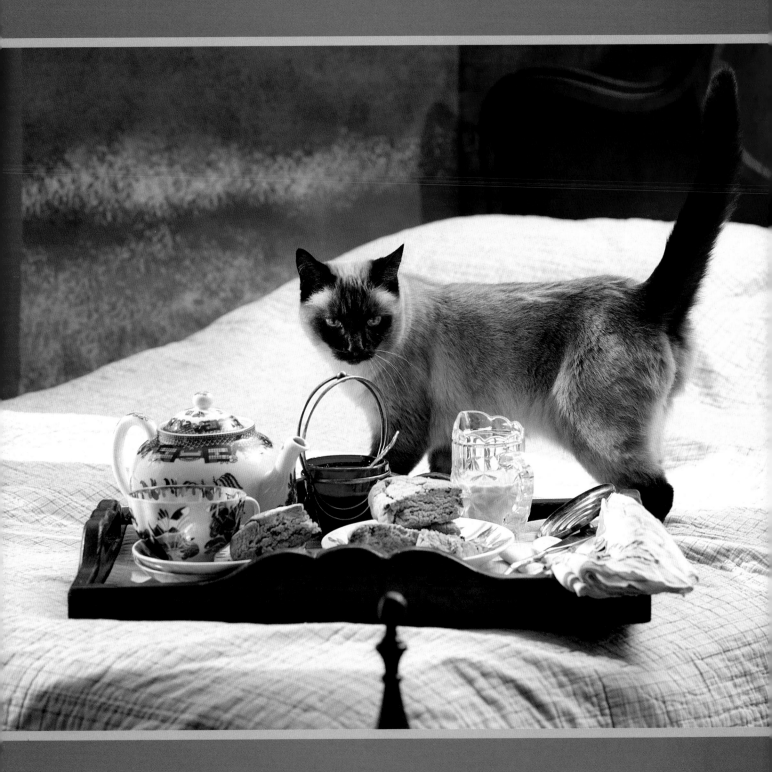

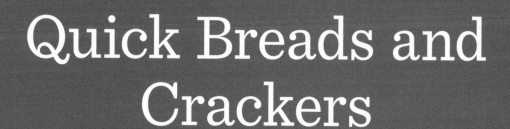

Quick Breads and Crackers

Quick breads are breads that don't use yeast to make them rise but instead usually use baking powder, baking soda, and/or eggs as a leavening agent. Of course, I use egg replacer and not bird eggs! And a cracker by definition is unleavened bread.

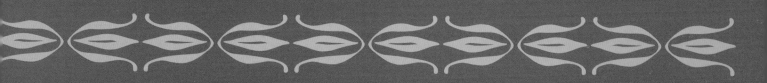

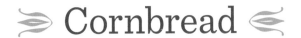 Cornbread

Here's the traditional recipe gone vegan.

1 tablespoon vegan margarine

1½ cups unsweetened coconut milk,
 soy milk, or almond milk

1½ tablespoons white vinegar

1 cup organic cornmeal

1 cup all-purpose flour

¼ cup sugar, or less to taste

¾ teaspoon salt

1 teaspoon baking powder

½ teaspoon baking soda

2 tablespoons safflower oil or canola oil

Preheat the oven to 425°F. Grease a 9-inch square baking dish with the margarine.

In a small bowl, combine the coconut milk and vinegar and let stand.

Place the cornmeal, flour, sugar, salt, baking powder, and baking soda in a large bowl and mix well. Add the coconut milk mixture and the safflower oil to the dry ingredients and stir just until blended, taking care not to overmix. Pour the batter into the prepared baking dish and bake for 25 to 30 minutes, or until a toothpick inserted into the center comes out clean.

SERVES 12

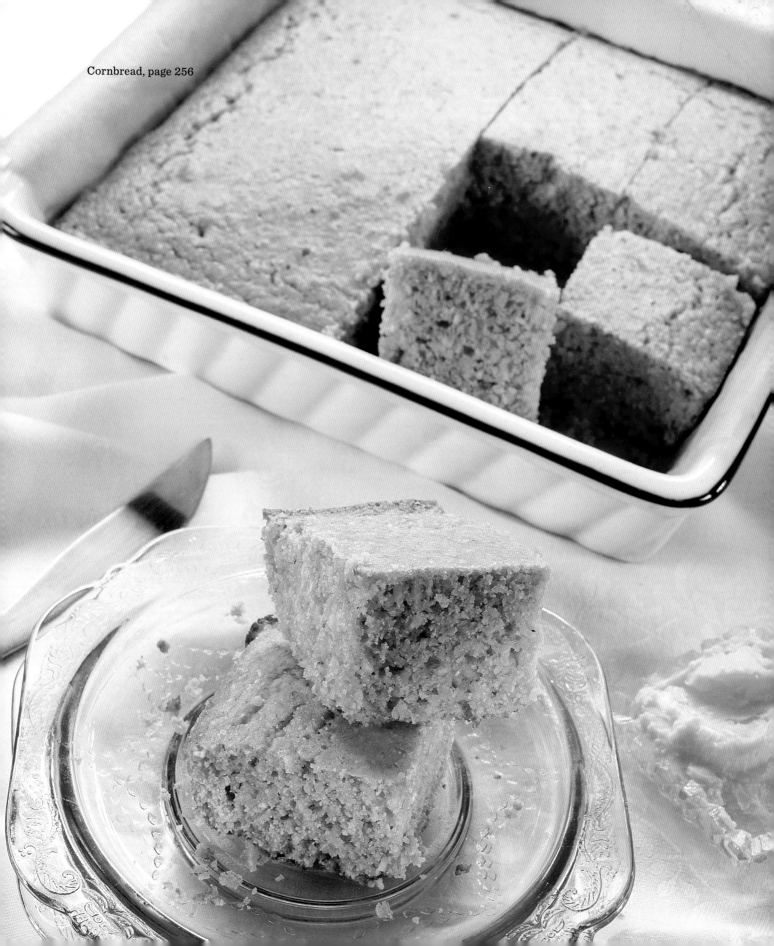

Cornbread, page 256

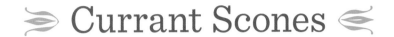

Currant Scones

Currant scones are always current.

1¾ cups all-purpose flour

2¼ teaspoons baking powder

1 tablespoon sugar

4 tablespoons (½ stick) cold vegan
    margarine or vegan shortening

¼ cup currants

⅓ cup soy milk

Preheat the oven to 425°F. Grease a 12 x 14-inch baking sheet and set aside.

In a large bowl, place the flour, baking powder, and sugar and mix well. Using two knives or a pastry cutter, cut in the margarine. In a small bowl, mix the currants and milk, then add to the flour mixture, combining with as few strokes as possible.

Gather and pat the batter down gently into a 6-inch-diameter circle on a floured board. Cut the circle like a pie into 6 wedges. Separate the wedges and place them on the prepared baking sheet. Bake for 15 to 20 minutes, until golden.

MAKES 6 SCONES

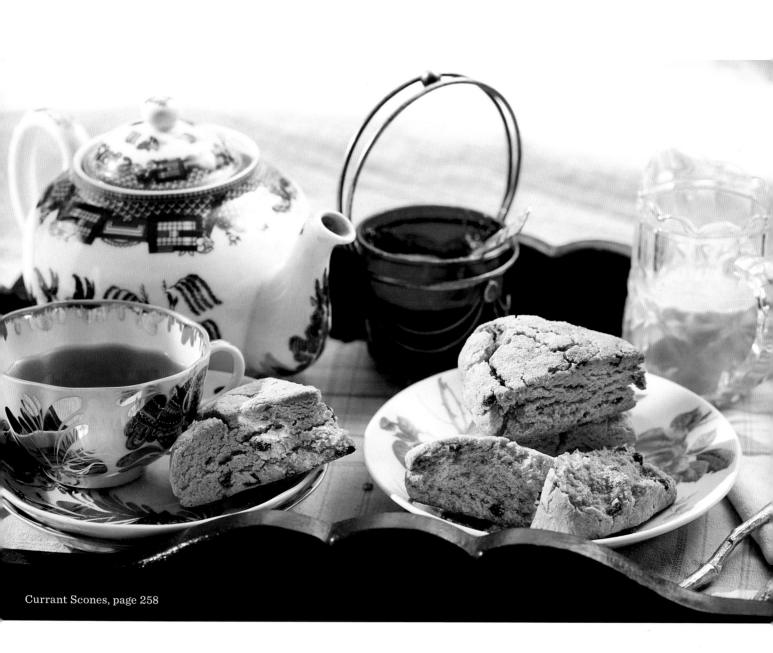

Currant Scones, page 258

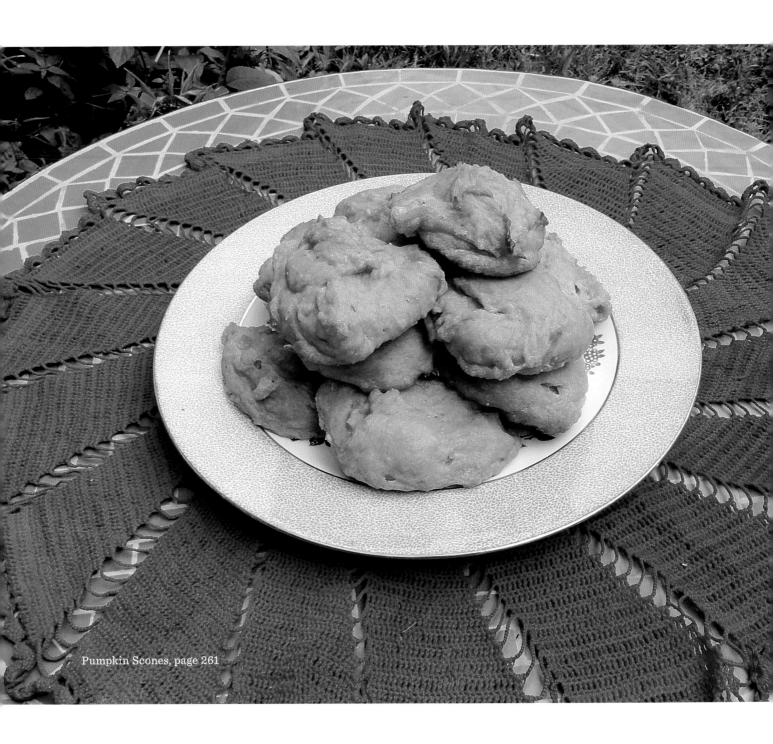

Pumpkin Scones, page 261

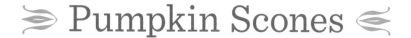

Pumpkin Scones

Pumpkin turns an ordinary scone into an autumn delight.

⅓ cup vegan margarine or tofu sour cream

One 15-ounce can pureed pumpkin, or 2 cups cooked and mashed fresh pumpkin

½ cup safflower oil or canola oil

2 tablespoons soy milk

1 teaspoon vanilla extract

1 tablespoon maple syrup

2 cups pastry flour

1 teaspoon baking powder

Pinch of salt

Preheat the oven to 400°F. Grease a 12 x 14-inch baking sheet and set aside.

In a medium bowl, place the margarine, pumpkin, safflower oil, soy milk, vanilla, and maple syrup and mix well, or use a blender. In a separate large bowl, stir together the flour, baking powder, and salt. Add the wet mixture to the dry ingredients and mix with a large spoon. The batter will be sticky. Using a large spoon, drop spoonfuls onto the prepared baking sheet and bake for 15 to 20 minutes, until brown on top and a toothpick inserted into the center comes out clean.

MAKES 10 TO 12 SCONES

⪼ Gopal's Gluten-Free ⪻ Crackers

My friend Gopal was looking for a protein-rich, gluten-free snack cracker. He knew that many vegans and raw-food enthusiasts make dehydrated crackers from flax meal, but he wanted a higher protein content, so he tried using red lentils, and this is the result.

1 cup red lentils

1¾ cups water

1 teaspoon ground cumin

½ tablespoon celery seeds

1 tablespoon onion powder

3 tablespoons dried chives

½ tablespoon poppy seeds

½ teaspoon chia seeds

1¼ teaspoons salt

¾ teaspoon freshly ground black pepper

½ teaspoon xanthan gum

2 tablespoons ground flax meal

Grease a 12 x 14-inch baking sheet and set aside.

In a large soup pot, place the lentils, rinse with cold water, then drain. Add the water and bring to a boil over high heat. Reduce the heat to low and simmer, covered, for 20 to 25 minutes, until almost all of the lentils have dissolved to the consistency of thick soup. Remove from the heat and let the cooked lentils sit, covered, for at least 5 minutes. Preheat the oven to 200°F.

Place the cumin, celery seeds, onion powder, chives, poppy seeds, chia seeds, salt, pepper, and xanthan gum in a medium bowl and whisk until well mixed. Add the mixture to the cooked lentils and mix well.

Taste and adjust the seasonings, particularly the salt and pepper. Then mix in the flax meal. Taste and adjust the seasonings again.

Spread the batter on the prepared baking sheet, then place a piece of parchment paper (or a cut-open brown paper bag) on top of the batter and, using a rolling pin, roll the batter so that it becomes even. Score the batter with a "butter" knife into 1-inch squares. Bake for 5 hours, until the crackers are crisp.

These crackers can also be made in a dehydrator if you have one. Lightly oil a dehydrator tray and spread the batter evenly on it (an offset spatula works best for this). Score the batter into cracker-size pieces (if you are multiplying the recipe and using more than one tray, it is best to wait until all the batter is spread on all the trays before scoring in case it is necessary to add more batter to some trays). Dehydrate the crackers at 115°F for 10 hours, then gently turn the crackers over and dehydrate for another 5 or 6 hours, until they reach the desired consistency. You may need to adjust the amount of dehydration time or even the temperature, depending on your dehydrator, the size of the tray, and the thickness of the batter on the tray. Also, reducing the time somewhat or using a lower temperature will result in denser crackers; increasing the time and/or temperature will result in crisper, crunchier crackers.

MAKES APPROXIMATELY 150 SMALL CRACKERS

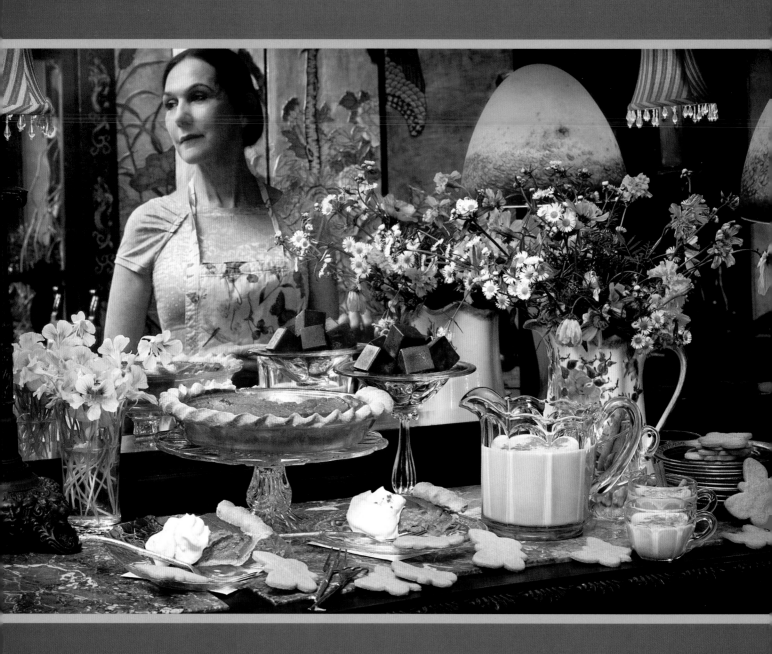

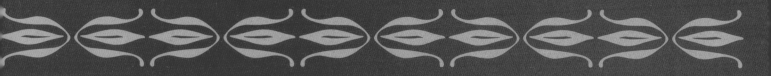

Desserts

A dessert is a sweet dish traditionally served as a final course of a meal. It derives from a French word meaning "to clear the table." That's why it is usually served at the end of a meal. But in the café world it is a respected custom to order dessert all by itself or accompanied with a drink like tea or coffee.

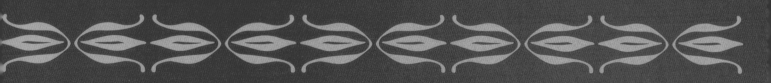

⇒ Sharon's Amazing ⇐ Chocolate Mousse

I worked for three years to arrive at what I think is a perfect formula; you be the judge.

One 14-ounce package extra-firm tofu

One 14-ounce package firm tofu

Pinch of salt

⅓ cup maple syrup or agave

10 ounces canned coconut milk

3 tablespoons vanilla extract

2 tablespoons unsweetened cocoa
     powder

2 tablespoons raw cacao powder

One 9-ounce bag vegan chocolate chips

2 tablespoons coconut oil

Simple Whipped Cream Topping (page
     295), optional

In the bowl of a food processor, place the tofu and salt and process until smooth. Add the maple syrup, coconut milk, vanilla, cocoa powder, and cacao powder and blend again until smooth.

In a double boiler, melt the chocolate chips and coconut oil. Add the melted mixture to the food processor and thoroughly blend.

Transfer the mixture to a large bowl, using a spatula to scrape it all out. Using a hand mixer, whip the mixture at high speed for 3 to 5 minutes to lighten it and add more air. Spoon into serving cups or shallow crystal champagne glasses and refrigerate for 1 to 2 hours, until cold. Garnish with a dollop of vegan whipped cream, if desired.

SERVES 15 TO 20, DEPENDING ON THE SIZE OF THE SERVING CUPS

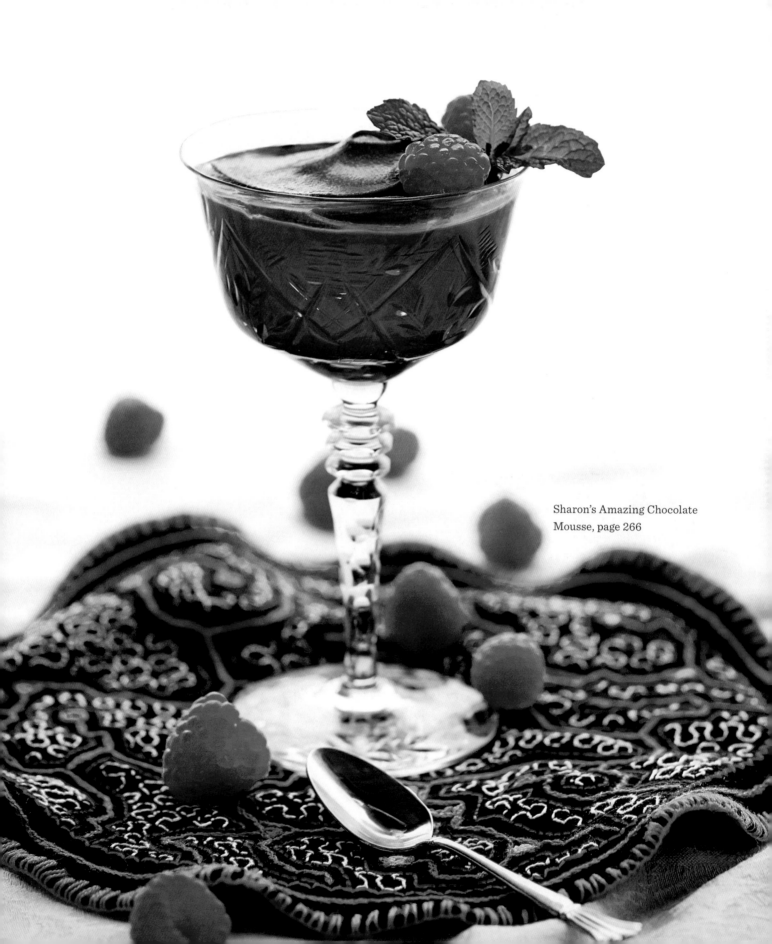

Sharon's Amazing Chocolate
Mousse, page 266

❧ Raw, Soy-Free ❧ Chocolate Pudding

Here's a delectable chocolate pudding that requires no cooking.

2 ripe avocados, peeled, with pits
   removed

2 tablespoons cacao powder

2 tablespoons agave

1 tablespoon vanilla extract

Pinch of salt

In the bowl of a food processor, place the avocados, cacao powder, agave, vanilla, and salt and process until very smooth. Pour into small individual dessert cups and refrigerate for 1 to 2 hours, until chilled.

SERVES 4

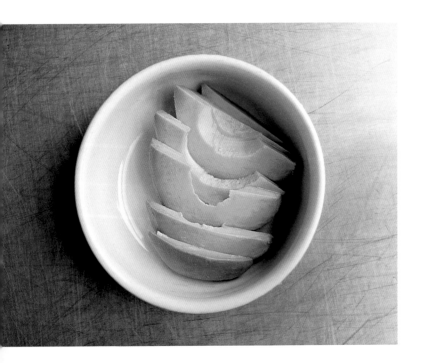

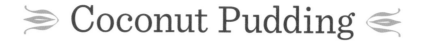

Coconut Pudding

Many people say that orchids have no smell, yet vanilla, the most popular flavoring, comes from an orchid. Vanilla enhances the delicate flavor of the coconut.

One 14-ounce package silken tofu

10 ounces canned coconut milk

¼ cup agave

1 teaspoon vanilla extract

½ cup shredded coconut

In the bowl of a food processor, place the tofu, coconut milk, agave, and vanilla and process until creamy. Transfer the blended ingredients to a large bowl and stir in the shredded coconut. Pour into dessert cups and refrigerate for at least 1 hour, until chilled.

SERVES 12

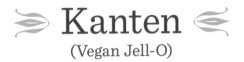

Kanten

(Vegan Jell-O)

Jell-O is made from gelatin—cow hooves and other animal by-products—yuck!
Here's a yummy vegan version that's been used in Japanese cuisine for many years.
The key ingredient is agar-agar, a type of tasteless seaweed that jells like gelatin.

4 cups apple juice

¼ cup agar-agar flakes

1 banana, thinly sliced

Simple Whipped Cream Topping
(page 295), optional

In a medium saucepan, place the apple juice and agar-agar, then bring to a boil over high heat and boil for 2 minutes, stirring continuously. Reduce the heat to low and simmer for 5 minutes to make sure the agar-agar is thoroughly dissolved.

Meanwhile, place the banana slices in individual serving cups. Pour the apple juice mixture over the bananas. Refrigerate for at least 1 hour, until chilled. Serve with a generous dollop of Simple Whipped Cream Topping, if desired.

VARIATION

Experiment by substituting coconut milk, tomato juice, or peach or other fruit juice for the apple juice, and substitute tomatoes or peaches, berries, or other fruits for the banana.

SERVES 12

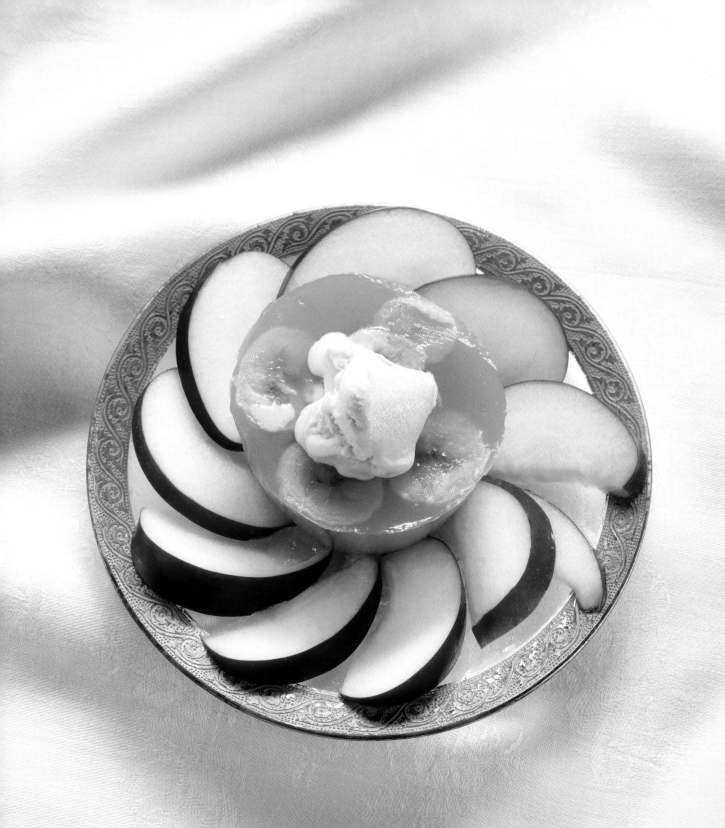

Kanten, page 270

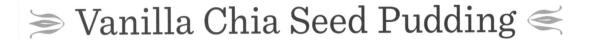 Vanilla Chia Seed Pudding

Simply blue and amazing!

3 cups almond milk, soy milk, or
coconut milk

1 cup chia seeds

1 teaspoon vanilla extract

1 tablespoon agave or maple syrup (use
more or less to taste)

In a large jar, place the almond milk, chia seeds, vanilla, and agave and shake vigorously until the ingredients are well mixed. The chia seeds will expand and become gelatinous but will remain whole. Pour the beautiful light blue pudding into small dessert cups and refrigerate for 1 to 2 hours, until chilled.

SERVES 12

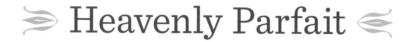 Heavenly Parfait

This dessert is a light, melt-in-your mouth confection.

4 cups apple juice, pear juice, or
pineapple juice

¼ cup agar-agar flakes

3 cups coconut milk

1 cup chia seeds

1 teaspoon vanilla extract

1 tablespoon agave or maple syrup (use
more or less to taste)

In a medium saucepan, place the apple juice and agar-agar and bring to a boil over high heat. Boil for 2 minutes, stirring continuously, then reduce the heat to low and simmer for 5 minutes, making sure the agar-agar is completely dissolved. Pour the kanten mixture into dessert bowls or parfait glasses and refrigerate for 1 hour.

Meanwhile, in a large jar, place the coconut milk, chia seeds, vanilla, and agave and shake vigorously until the ingredients are well mixed.

Take the kanten out of the refrigerator and spoon the chia seed pudding on top. Refrigerate for 1 hour more.

SERVES 12

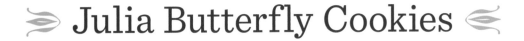 Julia Butterfly Cookies

To protest logging, my friend Julia Butterfly Hill lived in a fifteen-hundred-year-old redwood tree for more than two years. She says that when she came down from the tree, she was transformed, like a caterpillar morphing into a butterfly. My nephew and I wanted to bake cookies one day and we found a cookie cutter in the shape of a butterfly. Because we're both big fans of Julia, when he asked what kind of cookies we were going to make, I said, "Julia Butterfly cookies, of course!" Eat these cookies in or under a tree and send blessings to Julia!

½ pound (2 sticks) vegan margarine

1 cup sugar

3 cups all-purpose flour

2 teaspoons aluminum-free baking powder

1½ teaspoons powdered egg replacer

2 tablespoons water, plus more as needed

1 teaspoon vanilla extract

Preheat the oven to 400°F.

In a large bowl, cream the margarine and sugar. In a medium bowl, mix the flour and baking powder. In a separate, small bowl, using a whisk, beat the egg replacer with the water. Add the egg replacer and vanilla to the creamed margarine and sugar and stir to combine. Add the dry ingredients to the wet ingredients a little at a time and mix, adding a little water if needed. The dough should be very stiff.

Roll out the dough on a floured surface to a ¼-inch thickness. Using a butterfly-shaped cookie cutter dipped in flour, cut out the shapes. Place the cookies on an ungreased 12 x 14-inch baking sheet and bake for about 8 minutes, until golden brown. Remove the baking sheet from the oven and transfer the cookies to a wire rack to cool.

MAKES ABOUT 20 COOKIES

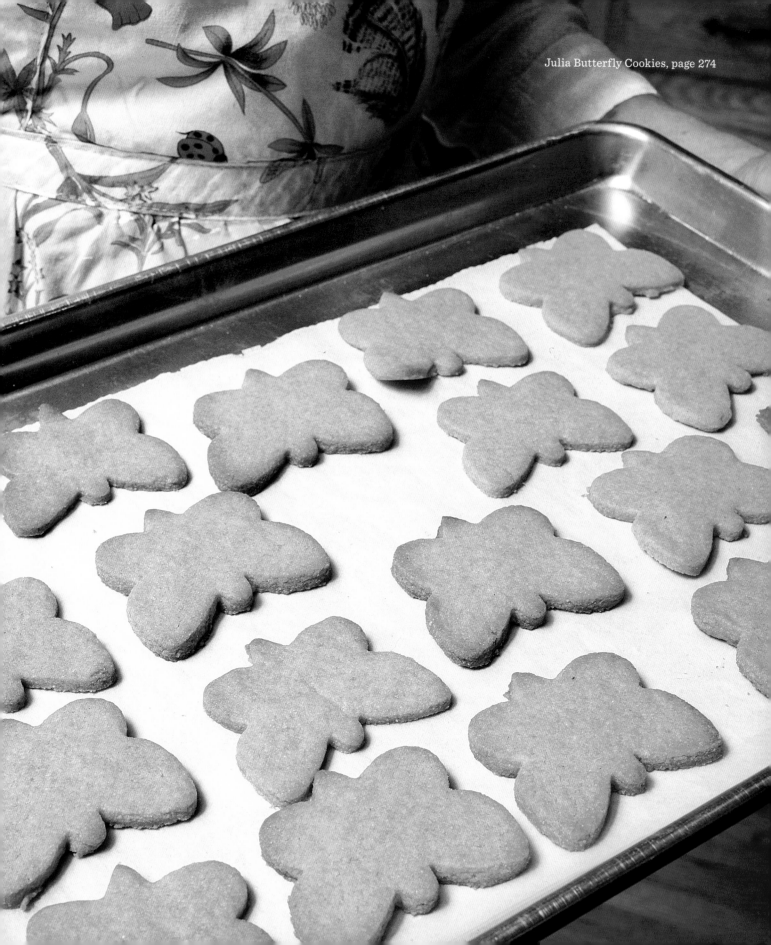
Julia Butterfly Cookies, page 274

⇌ Gingerbread Cookies ⇌

These cookies are great for Christmastime—or anytime.

½ pound (2 sticks) vegan margarine, at
    room temperature, plus more for
    greasing the baking sheet
1 cup sugar
Egg replacer equivalent of 1 egg
1 cup molasses
2 tablespoons cider vinegar

5 cups all-purpose flour
½ teaspoon salt
1½ teaspoons baking soda
1 tablespoon ground ginger
1¼ teaspoons ground cinnamon
1 teaspoon ground cloves
1 recipe Vanilla Sugar Icing (page 292)

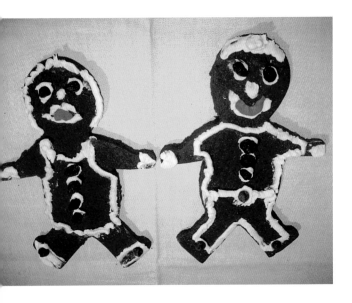

In a large bowl, cream the margarine and sugar. Mix in the egg replacer, molasses, and vinegar and set aside.

In a medium bowl, sift together the flour, salt, baking soda, ginger, cinnamon, and cloves. Add the dry ingredients to the wet ingredients and mix well.

Divide the dough into 3 equal balls, wrap tightly in plastic wrap or damp dishcloths, and refrigerate for at least 3 hours or overnight.

Preheat the oven to 375°F. Lightly grease a 12 x 14-inch baking sheet with vegan margarine and set aside.

Remove the dough from the refrigerator and let it sit for 5 minutes, until it is soft enough to roll. Using a rolling pin, roll each ball of dough out on a floured surface to a ¼-inch thickness. If the dough is too crumbly, mix a very little bit of water into the dough to help it to stick together. Using a cookie cutter, cut the dough into shapes and arrange them on the prepared baking sheet. For a traditional gingerbread man or woman, use a human-shaped cutter, but don't limit yourself—gingerbread cats and dogs and cows and chickens are people too and just as tasty and so much kinder than eating the real thing. Trees, houses, and geometric shapes also make great cookies. Bake for 6 to 8 minutes, or until the edges are brown.

Remove from the oven, cool for 5 minutes on the baking sheet, then transfer to a wire rack to cool completely. While the cookies are cooling, make the icing. When the cookies are cool, fill a pastry bag with the icing and, using a star tip, decorate the cookies.

Decorating options: Apply the frosting as an outline to suggest clothes or cover the whole surface of the cookie with the frosting. Press into the frosting raisins, currants, chocolate chips, or nuts to form eyes, mouth, nose, buttons, etc.

MAKES 12 LARGE (8-INCH) COOKIES

⋙ Chocolate Ice Cream Cake ⋘

Here is a cake-size, vegan ice cream sandwich.

1¾ cups pastry flour, plus more for dusting the pans

2 cups sugar

¾ cup unsweetened cocoa powder

1½ teaspoons baking soda

1½ teaspoons baking powder

1 teaspoon salt

2 teaspoons powdered egg replacer, dissolved in ¼ cup water

½ cup water

1 cup soy milk or almond milk

½ cup vegetable oil

2 teaspoons vanilla extract

Warm water, as needed

1 pint vanilla or chocolate vegan ice cream

Preheat the oven to 350°F. Grease the bottoms and sides of two 9-inch square cake pans with vegan margarine, then dust with flour; set aside.

In a large bowl, place the flour, sugar, cocoa powder, baking soda, baking powder, and salt and mix well. In another large bowl, whisk the dissolved egg replacer until frothy. Add the dry ingredients, soy milk, vegetable oil, and vanilla and blend with a mixer, adding warm water as needed (up to ½ cup) to yield a thin batter.

Divide the batter between the prepared cake pans and bake for 35 to 40 minutes, until a toothpick or "butter" knife inserted into the center comes out clean. Place the pans on wire racks until completely cooled. Then remove one cake from the cake pan and place it on a freezer-proof plate. Soften the ice cream by letting it stand at room temperature for 5 minutes, then spread the ice cream about 1 inch thick over the top of the cake. Remove the other cake from the cake pan and

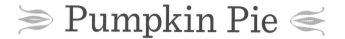

Pumpkin Pie

Traditionally eggs hold a pumpkin pie together, but the combination of tofu and cornstarch works just as well.

14 ounces firm tofu

Two 15-ounce cans pureed pumpkin

1 cup firmly packed dark brown sugar

¼ cup melted coconut oil

2 tablespoons molasses

¼ cup organic non-GMO cornstarch

1½ teaspoons ground cinnamon

2 teaspoons vanilla extract

½ teaspoon salt

½ teaspoon ground nutmeg

¼ teaspoon ground cloves

¼ teaspoon ground ginger

¼ teaspoon ground allspice

½ recipe Piecrust (page 286)

Simple Whipped Cream Topping
  (page 295)

Preheat the oven to 350°F.

In the bowl of a food processor, place the tofu, pumpkin, brown sugar, coconut oil, molasses, cornstarch, cinnamon, vanilla, salt, nutmeg, cloves, ginger, and allspice and process until creamy. Pour the filling into the piecrust and bake for 1 hour. Cool on a wire rack, then cover and refrigerate for at least 5 hours while the pie sets. Serve individual slices with a dollop of whipped cream.

SERVES 8 TO 12

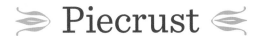

Piecrust

Many people maintain that you can't make a flaky piecrust without butter. I beg to differ. If you want a flaky crust, make sure that all of the ingredients are super cold. Even so, the secret ingredient to this crust is the vinegar, which helps prevent the formation of gluten, which would make the crust tough. This recipe makes a double crust. If you need only a single crust, as is the case for a pumpkin pie, then halve the recipe. As for the pie pan, I find that glass pans are best because they conduct the heat more evenly than ceramic or metal pans.

8 tablespoons (1 stick) vegan margarine, very cold
8 tablespoons (1 stick) vegan shortening, very cold
2½ cups pastry flour, plus more for dusting
½ teaspoon salt
3 tablespoons sugar
4 to 6 tablespoons ice water
1 tablespoon apple cider vinegar, very cold
Vegetable oil, for greasing the pie pan

Cut the sticks of margarine and shortening into ½ tablespoon chunks and place in the refrigerator or freezer for at least 30 minutes, until very cold.

While the margarine and shortening are chilling, sift the flour and salt into a large bowl, then mix in the sugar. Using a pastry cutter or two "butter" knives, cut in the margarine and shortening ½ tablespoon at a time until the mixture looks pebbly.

In a small cup, combine 4 tablespoons of the ice water and the vinegar. Add the vinegar mixture to the batter slowly, 1 teaspoon at a time, using the pastry cutter or two knives to mix after each addition. With your hands, knead the dough until it comes together into a ball, adding a bit more ice water if necessary to get the dough to hold together. For a flaky crust, the dough should look rather rough, not like a dense solid mass. Wrap the dough tightly in plastic wrap and refrigerate it for at least 30 minutes before rolling.

When ready to roll, place the dough on a floured cutting board and, using a floured rolling pin, roll the dough into a large circle. Place a 9-inch pie pan on top of the dough and, using a knife, cut a large dough circle, approximately 1 inch larger than the pan. Reserve any extra dough. Note: Extra dough can be kept in the refrigerator for up to a week, if it is tightly covered.

Grease and flour the bottom and sides of the pie pan, then press the dough into the pan with your fingers, making sure that the dough covers the bottom and sides of the pan evenly. Using your thumb and forefinger, pinch the dough at 1-inch intervals at the top edge of the pie pan, or use a fork to make depressions around the top edge.

Fill the uncooked piecrust with the filling of your choice, then use the rest of the dough to make a cover for the pie. Using a floured rolling pin, roll out the reserved dough into a circle and lay it on top of the pie, pinching the edges together with the bottom layer of dough, or cut the dough into strips and "weave" them across the top of the filling, pressing the edges into the dough on the sides.

VARIATION

Alternatively, use the rest of the dough to make simple sugar cookies. Add $\frac{1}{8}$ cup of sugar and 1 teaspoon of vanilla extract or almond extract and knead the dough thoroughly. Place on a floured cutting board and roll out the dough with a floured rolling pin. Cut the dough into shapes using a cookie cutter, then place the cookies on a lightly greased baking sheet and bake at 425°F for about 10 minutes, until golden brown. Remove the cookies from the oven and transfer to a wire rack to cool.

MAKES TWO 9-INCH PIE SHELLS OR ONE 9-INCH COVERED PIECRUST

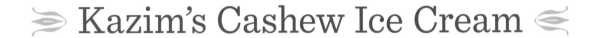 Kazim's Cashew Ice Cream

Kazim Ali, a poet friend of mine, developed this ice cream as a dessert poem for me.

1 cup cashews

2 cups soy milk, almond milk, or
    coconut milk

1 avocado, peeled and pitted

½ cup maple syrup or agave

¼ cup peanut butter or almond butter

1 tablespoon vanilla extract

1 teaspoon salt

¼ cup unsweetened cocoa
    powder

Soak the cashews in 1½ cups water for at least 4 hours or overnight. Drain.

In the bowl of a food processor or in a blender jar, place the cashews, soy milk, avocado, maple syrup, peanut butter, vanilla, salt, and cocoa powder and process or blend until creamy. Pour into a 1-quart container, cover, and let sit in the freezer at least 6 hours, until frozen.

SERVES 10 TO 12

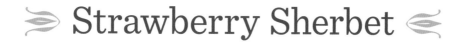 Strawberry Sherbet

I love this on a hot summer afternoon on my porch overlooking
the forest, especially when the berries come from my garden.

1 cup frozen strawberries (or substitute
blueberries or raspberries)

1 cup almond milk, soy milk, or coconut
milk

1 tablespoon vanilla extract

1 tablespoon agave

In the bowl of a food processor or in the blender jar of a heavy-duty blender, place the strawberries, almond milk, vanilla, and agave and process or blend until creamy. Pour into a 1-quart container and freeze, covered, for at least 6 hours.

SERVES 1 TO 2

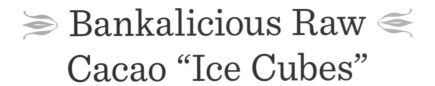 Bankalicious Raw Cacao "Ice Cubes"

This is a staple at my home when my dear friend Banka comes to visit in August.

One 8-ounce jar raw coconut butter, peanut butter, almond butter, cashew butter, or cacao butter

One 8-ounce jar coconut oil

1 cup cacao powder

¼ cup agave or coconut nectar

1 tablespoon vanilla extract

1 or 2 pinches of salt

Pour hot water into a large bowl and place the glass jars of the coconut butter and coconut oil in it. The butter will become creamy and the oil will become liquid. Empty the contents of both jars into a large bowl and add the cacao powder, agave, vanilla, and salt. Stir in unconditional love, patience, compassion, wildness, and wisdom. Pour into ice cube trays or molds and freeze for at least 2 hours.

VARIATIONS

- Add 1 teaspoon cayenne, ground cardamom, or ground ginger.
- Add 1 to 2 drops lavender oil.
- Add ¼ cup cacao nibs, which will give the confection a crunch.

MAKES APPROXIMATELY 24 CUBES

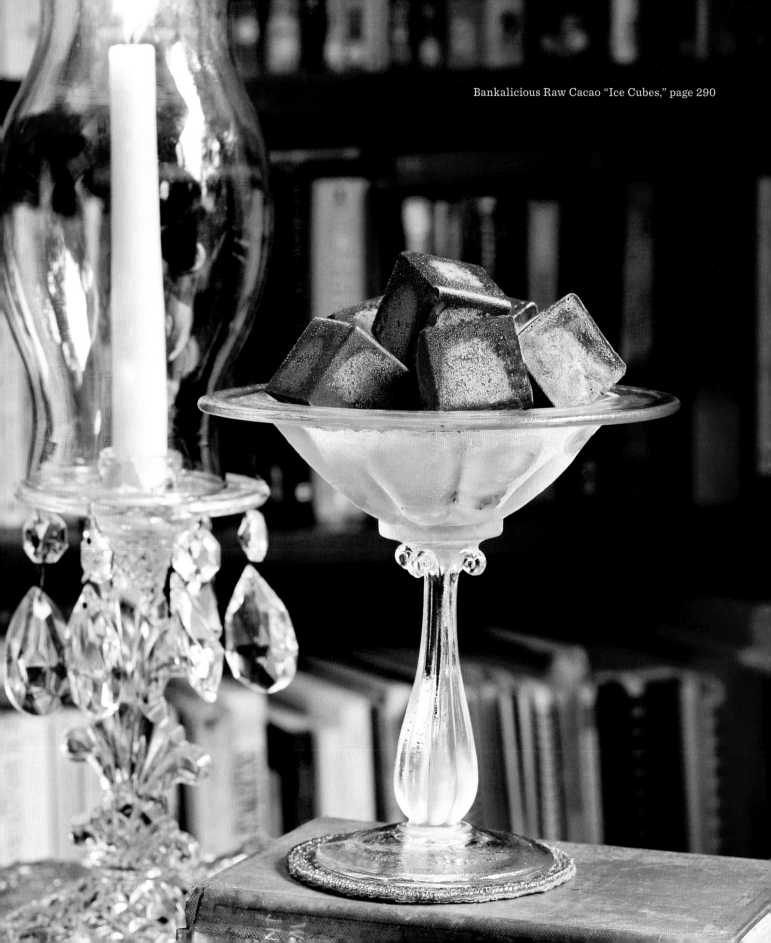

Bankalicious Raw Cacao "Ice Cubes," page 290

Vanilla Sugar Icing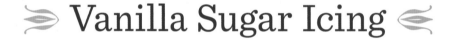

8 tablespoons (1 stick) vegan margarine,
    at room temperature
2 cups confectioners' sugar

1 teaspoon vanilla extract
1½ teaspoons vanilla soy milk

In a large bowl, place the margarine and cream using a hand mixer. Add the sugar, vanilla, and soy milk and mix on medium speed until thoroughly combined. The icing should be stiff. Store in a tightly covered container in the refrigerator until ready to use. You may have to rewhip the icing before spreading it on a cake.

MAKES ENOUGH TO FROST ONE 9-INCH LAYER CAKE OR

8 LARGE GINGERBREAD COOKIES

⋐ Chocolate Obsession ⋑ Frosting

8 tablespoons (1 stick) vegan margarine, at room temperature

2½ cups confectioners' sugar

⅓ cup unsweetened cocoa powder

1 teaspoon vanilla extract

3 to 4 tablespoons soy milk, plus more as needed

In a large bowl, place the margarine and cream until smooth using a hand mixer. Add the sugar, cocoa powder, vanilla, and soy milk and mix on medium speed until thoroughly combined. Raise the speed to high and mix for about 3 minutes, until the frosting is fluffy and stiff. Store in a tightly covered container in the refrigerator until ready to use. You may have to rewhip the frosting before using.

MAKES ENOUGH TO FROST ONE 9-INCH CAKE

⋐ Faux Cream Cheese Icing ⋑

1 cup confectioners' sugar

One 8-ounce package vegan cream cheese, cold

1 teaspoon vanilla extract

In a large bowl, using an electric mixer set on medium speed, break up the sugar to remove lumps, then add the cream cheese and vanilla and mix well.

VARIATION

For a chocolate version, add 3 tablespoons unsweetened cocoa powder and mix well.

MAKES ENOUGH TO FROST ONE 9-INCH CAKE

⮜ Sugar-Free Icing ⮞

4 ounces dried dates

2 ounces dried apricots

¼ cup coconut oil, or 4 tablespoons (½ stick) vegan margarine

Flavor the icing with one of these options:

1 tablespoon vanilla extract

1 tablespoon unsweetened cocoa powder

Juice from 1 lemon, plus 2 tablespoons grated zest

Juice from 1 orange, plus 2 tablespoons grated zest

In a small bowl, soak the dates and apricots in water to cover until they are soft. Or, in a small saucepan, place the dates and apricots and enough water to cover. Cook over low heat until the apricots and dates are soft, then allow them to cool.

Drain the fruit, reserving the soaking water. In the bowl of a food processor or blender, place the fruit and process well, gradually adding the coconut oil and whatever flavoring you are using. Add some soaking water if needed to yield a smooth consistency.

Place the icing in the refrigerator for 2 to 3 hours, until the consistency is stiff and the icing is cold.

MAKES ENOUGH TO FROST ONE 9-INCH CAKE

⇒ Simple Whipped ⇐ Cream Topping

This topping is great on Pumpkin Pie (page 285), Sharon's Amazing Chocolate
Mousse (page 266), or Kanten (Vegan Jell-O) (page 270). The secret
is to use full-fat coconut milk, and it must be very cold.

One 10-ounce can coconut milk
1 teaspoon vanilla extract
2 tablespoons confectioners' sugar

Place the can of coconut milk in the refrigerator overnight. When ready to whip, remove the can from the refrigerator and gently turn it upside down, taking care not to shake it. Open the can and pour the separated liquid into a small container and set aside for use in any other dish, such as smoothies, soups, etc. It should be about ½ cup. Using a spatula, scoop out the solidified "cream" and place the cream, vanilla, and sugar in a small bowl, then mix using a hand whisk or an electric mixer set on high speed until the topping looks fluffy, like whipped cream. Chill in the refrigerator for about 2 hours, until the mixture is firm.

MAKES 1 CUP

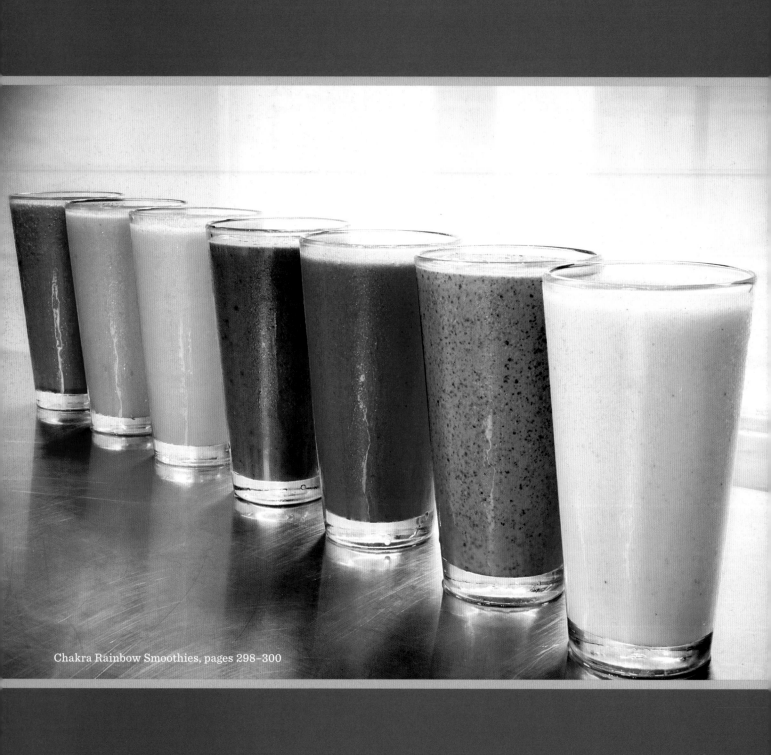

Chakra Rainbow Smoothies, pages 298–300

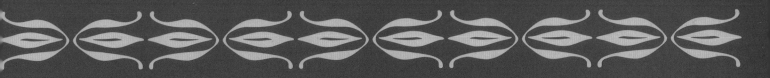

Smoothies

Smoothies are like liquid desserts, but they tend to be more nutritious than desserts, so they can be eaten as a light meal on their own. I extend the definition of smoothie to include "milk" shakes and eggnog.

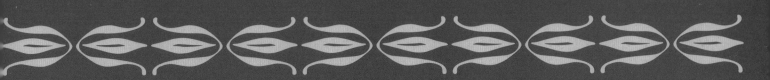

⇒ Chakra Rainbow ⇐ Smoothies

According to yogic tradition, each of us has a rainbow inside corresponding to seven energy centers known as chakras. When the chakras are at the height of their expression, they exude virtues and colors that radiate as auras around us. Choose your smoothie according to the virtue and color you wish to embody.

For each of these smoothies, in the blender jar of a heavy-duty blender place all the ingredients and blend until smooth but thick. Fills one 14-ounce glass.

ENLIGHTENMENT SMOOTHIE
(Sahasrara, Crown Chakra—White)

1 cup coconut water

2 tablespoons agave

1 tablespoon finely chopped peeled fresh ginger

1 cup frozen banana slices

WISDOM SMOOTHIE
(Ajña, Third Eye Chakra—Purple)

1 cup coconut water

1 teaspoon vanilla extract

¼ cup frozen açaí

1 cup frozen banana slices

TRUTH SMOOTHIE
(Vishuddha, Throat Chakra—Blue)

1 cup almond milk

2 tablespoons agave

1 tablespoon almond butter

½ cup frozen blueberries

½ cup frozen strawberries

LOVE SMOOTHIE
(Anahata, Heart Chakra—Green)

1 cup almond milk

1 cup frozen banana slices

2 leaves kale

2 teaspoons spirulina powder

1 medjool date, pitted and diced

CONFIDENCE SMOOTHIE
(Manipura, Power Chakra—Yellow)

1 cup coconut water

2 tablespoons agave

2 tablespoons fresh lemon juice

1 cup frozen mango slices

SEXY SMOOTHIE
(Swadishthana, Sexual/Creative Chakra—Orange)

1 cup orange juice

½ cup mango slices

½ cup strawberry slices

STABILITY SMOOTHIE
(Muladhara, Root Chakra—Red)

1 cup coconut water

1 tablespoon unsweetened cocoa
   powder

¼ cup frozen cherries

½ cup frozen strawberries

½ cup frozen raspberries

2 teaspoons agave

Vegan Chocolate "Milk" Shake

This "milk" shake is not too sweet or rich but is still more than satisfying.

1 cup soy milk, almond milk, or coconut milk

2 tablespoons full-fat canned coconut milk

1 tablespoon unsweetened cocoa powder

1 teaspoon cacao powder

2 teaspoons agave

¼ teaspoon vanilla extract

12 ice cubes

In a blender, place the soy milk, coconut milk, cocoa powder, cacao powder, agave, vanilla, and ice cubes and blend until thick and frothy.

SERVES 1

Vegan Eggnog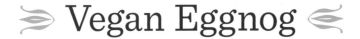

Here's an eggnog without the egg or the nog. The word *eggnog* is said to derive from "egg 'n grog," referring to the whiskey or rum that was the base of this English holiday treat made with eggs, milk, and sugar.

4 cups soy milk

1 ounce instant vegan vanilla pudding powder

One 10- to 15-ounce can coconut milk

2 tablespoons confectioners' sugar

2 teaspoons vanilla extract

½ teaspoon salt

¼ teaspoon ground nutmeg

¼ teaspoon ground cinnamon

In a medium bowl, place 2 cups of the soy milk and the instant pudding and stir well until thickened. Add the remaining 2 cups soy milk, coconut milk, sugar, vanilla, salt, and nutmeg and mix well. Refrigerate for at least 2 hours or overnight. Sprinkle with the cinnamon before serving.

SERVES 10 TO 12

WISDOM ~ ACAI, BANANA,
VANILLA EXTRACT. + COCONUT WATER.

TRUTH ~ BLUEBERRIES, ALMOND
BUTTER, BANANA, AGAVE, SOY MILK 10.50

LOVE ~ MEDJOOL DATE, BANANA
SPIRULINA, KALE, + ALMOND MILK 11.50

CONFIDENT ~ MANGO, LEMON 9.50
JUICE, AGAVE NECTAR, + COCONUT WATER

SEXY ~ ORANGE JUICE, MANGO, 10
STRAWBERRY

ABUNDANT ~ CHERRY, STRAWBERRY 10
RASPBERRY, COCOA + COCONUT WATER

ADD VEGA PERFORMANCE PROTEIN $2

EXTRAS:
SPIRULINA $1.25   TO GO 25¢
GINGER $.75
DRESSINGS $1

HARVEST ~ GRA
APPLES, RAW WALNUTS,
SEEDS, + DRIED CRANBE

SIMPLE SALA
WITH CHERRY TOMATO
CARROTS   (GF)

DRESSINGS:
BALSAMIC VINA
CAESAR
CARROT GING
CHIMICHURR
MAPLE VINAIG
MUSTARD VIN
SPICY
URME

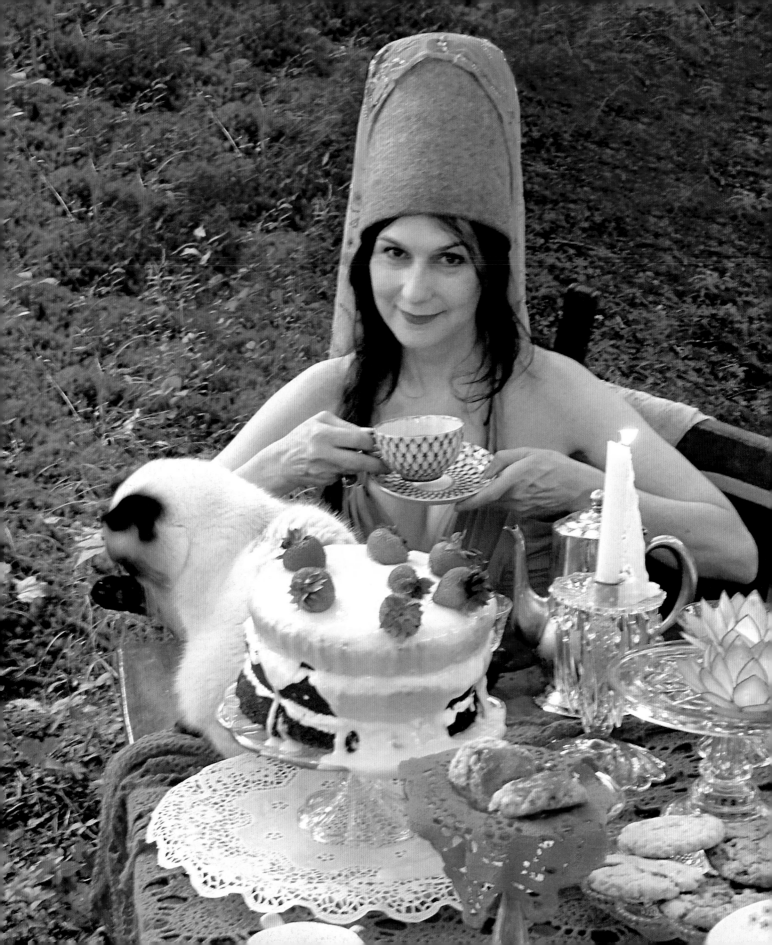

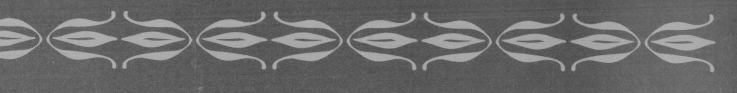

Tea and Other Hot Drinks

I personally have quite a fondness for tea. I love all kinds of tea: black, white, green, oolong, and herbal. To me, other drinks appear crass compared to the elegance of tea. Jivamuktea Café, with its own line of organic teas, was conceived as a platform to share the delights of tea with others.

To maintain the delicate flavor, tea should not be boiled but rather steeped. Because tea is made by infusing the leaves of the plant in hot water, tea is often called an infusion. Here's a simple guide to how to brew tea as an infusion: use 1 teaspoon loose tea for each 8-ounce cup, add boiling water, and steep for three minutes for white, green, and oolong; five minutes for black; and seven minutes for most herbal teas.

Some teas are not made with the leaves of a plant, nor are they steeped. Ginger and licorice tea are examples of this. They are made from the root of the ginger or licorice plant and are boiled to release the flavors. Flowers, like chamomile, hibiscus, and rose, can also make good tea by the infusion method. I could go on and on about tea but will leave that for another book. I'll share some recipes with you instead.

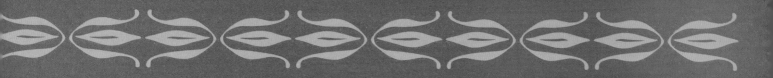

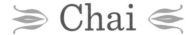 Chai

The Hindi word for tea is *chai*, so it is actually incorrect to say "chai tea," which literally means "tea tea." But nowadays when you order chai, it usually means masala or spiced tea. This type of chai has become quite popular and has been warmly embraced by yogis and so-called normal people everywhere. You can even find chai tea on the menus of many well-known coffeehouse chains throughout the world.

1 cardamom pod

2 black peppercorns

1 clove

½ teaspoon ground cinnamon

¼ teaspoon ground ginger

2 teaspoons loose Assam black tea

2 cups water

2 cups soy milk, almond milk, or
coconut milk

2 tablespoons sugar

¼ teaspoon vanilla extract

In a mortar, place the cardamom, peppercorns, and clove and crush using a pestle or the back of a spoon. In a tea ball, place the crushed spices, cinnamon, and ginger. In another tea ball, place the black tea.

In a medium saucepan, bring the water to a boil over high heat and add the tea ball that has the spices. Reduce the heat to medium-low and simmer for 5 minutes. Stir in the soy milk and sugar, raise the heat until the mixture is almost but not quite boiling, then add the tea ball containing the black tea. Turn off the heat, cover, and let steep for 5 minutes. Remove the two tea balls and stir in the vanilla. Serve this tea hot. If you need to reheat the tea, be careful not to bring it to a boil. If you don't have tea balls, then use a tea strainer to strain the tea into cups before serving.

SERVES 2 TO 4

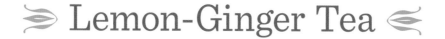 Lemon-Ginger Tea

Hot ginger tea on a cold day warms the body, brings clarity to the mind, and calms the soul. You can make a lot of this tea by doubling this recipe and storing it in the refrigerator. Reheat it when you crave another cup of this healing elixir.

One 1-inch piece fresh ginger root, peeled and finely chopped

4 cups water

2 tablespoons agave

2 tablespoons lemon juice

In a medium saucepan, place the ginger, add the water, and bring to a boil over high heat. Reduce the heat to medium and simmer for 15 minutes. Stir in the agave and lemon juice. To serve, pour through a tea strainer.

SERVES 2 TO 4

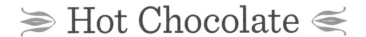 Hot Chocolate

This recipes tastes like cocoa with marshmallows.

1 cup water

3 tablespoons unsweetened cocoa
    powder

2 tablespoons sugar

¼ teaspoon salt, or less to taste

2 cups soy milk

½ teaspoon vanilla extract

Coconut milk, to garnish

In a small saucepan, place the water and bring to a boil. Reduce the heat to medium, add the cocoa powder, sugar, and salt, and simmer for about 1 minute, until dissolved. Add the soy milk, raise the heat, and bring the mixture to almost, but not quite, a boil. Turn off the heat and stir in the vanilla. Pour the chocolate into serving cups, then, holding a spoon of coconut milk over each cup, drizzle the coconut milk in a circular fashion over the chocolate. The result will be a marbleized white swirl in the dark chocolate.

SERVES 2

⋙ Italian Café–Style ⋘ Hot Chocolate

I have tried to replicate the experience of drinking hot chocolate in outdoor cafés in Rome and Florence, where it's served in small demitasse cups like espresso and traditionally without milk. If you're not used to drinking chocolate this way, you may find the taste slightly bitter. Feel free to sweeten as you like or even add a bit of soy milk to mellow the experience.

1 cup water

2 ounces nondairy semisweet chocolate chips

¼ teaspoon vanilla extract

Sugar and/or soy milk to taste, optional

In a small saucepan, place the water and bring to a boil. Add the chocolate chips and stir for 1 to 2 minutes, until dissolved. Stir in the vanilla and the sugar and/or soy milk to taste, if using, and pour into small cups.

SERVES 4

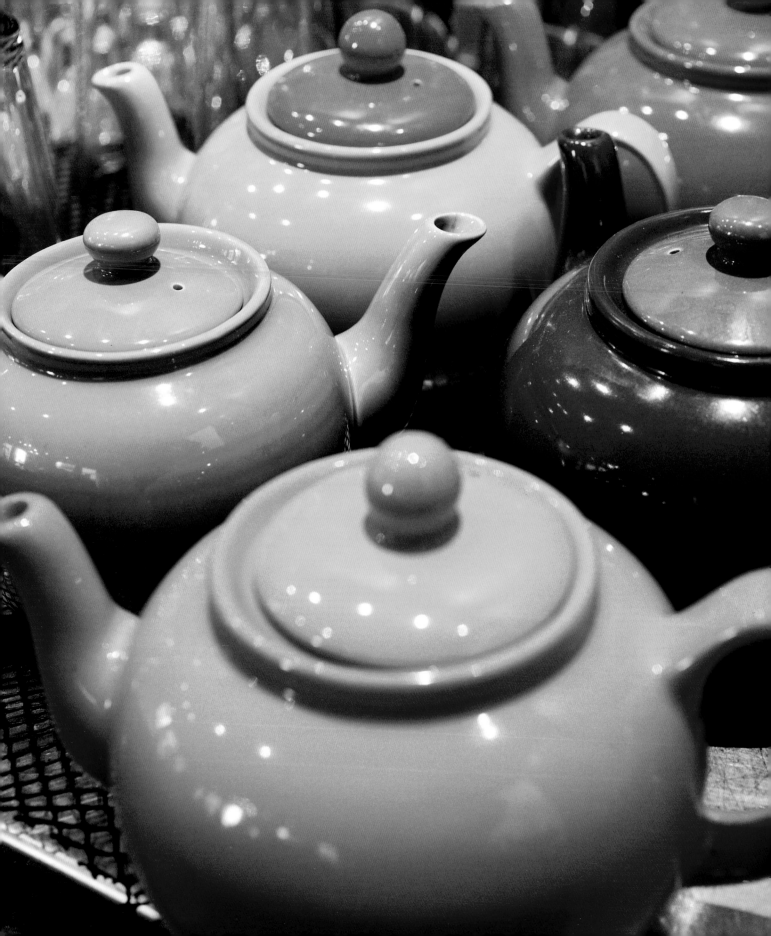

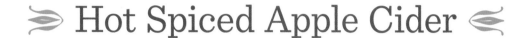 Hot Spiced Apple Cider

Perfect for winter holiday gatherings. The cranberries give
the cider a punchy tartness, as well as a pink glow.

½ gallon apple cider

4 cinnamon sticks

4 cloves

¼ teaspoon ground nutmeg

1 tablespoon agave, plus more to taste

½ cup fresh cranberries

1 teaspoon vanilla extract

In a medium saucepan, place the cider, cinnamon sticks, cloves, nutmeg, agave, and cranberries and bring to a boil over high heat. Reduce the heat to medium and simmer for 15 minutes. Add the vanilla and simmer for 1 more minute. Taste the cider. If it is too strong or too tart, add some water or some additional agave to taste.

SERVES 8 TO 16

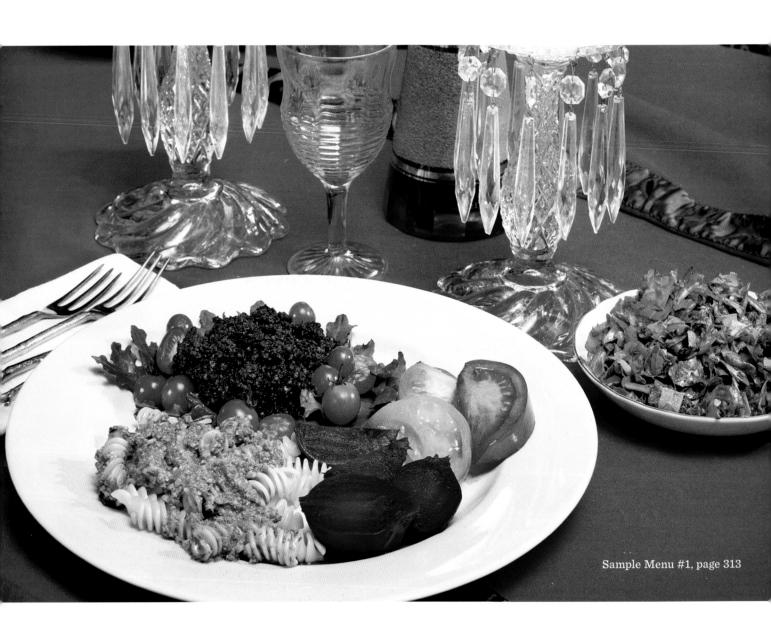

Sample Menu #1, page 313

30 Sample Menus

Try these menus for lunch or dinner.

1.

Pasta with Pesto (page 98), using rotini pasta

Spirulina Millet (page 180)

Simple Steamed Veggies (page 208): sliced beets

Green Leaves and Sweet Pepper Salad (page 122)

2.

Very Red Tomato and Beet Soup (page 53)

Flower Salad (page 121), with The Most Simple Dressing (page 152)

Simple Steamed Veggies (page 208): potatoes, zucchini, and winter squash

3.

Brown Rice (page 172)

Deluxe White Bean "Gravy" (page 193)

Simple Steamed Veggies (page 208): collard greens

Red Cabbage Coleslaw (page 137)

Cornbread (page 256)

4.

Savory Pumpkin Soup (page 81)

Simple Steamed Veggies (page 208): potatoes and green peas

Rosemary Seitan (page 197)

Arugula Salad (page 121), with The Most Simple Dressing (page 152)

5.

New England "Clam" Chowder (page 70)

Caesar Salad (page 128), with Caesar Dressing (page 157)

6.

Quick-and-Easy Cream of Tomato Soup (page 50)

Grilled Cheese (page 242)

7.

Country Vegetable Soup (page 73)

Caesar Salad (page 128), with Caesar Dressing (page 157)

"Poached Eggs" on Toast (page 232)

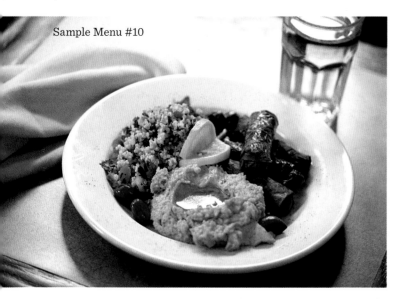
Sample Menu #10

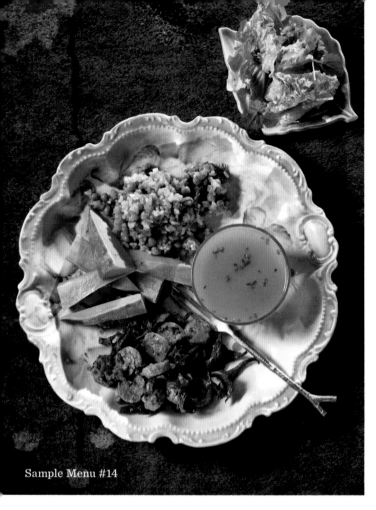

Sample Menu #14

16.

Red Lentil and Tomato Soup (page 63)

Simple Steamed Veggies (page 208): winter squash

Green Salad (page 118), with The Most Simple Dressing (page 152)

Spirulina Millet (page 180)

17.

Kabocha Squash Soup (page 55)

Spirulina Millet (page 180)

Simple Bean "Gravy" (page 192) using lima beans

Simple Steamed Veggies (page 208): cauliflower

Artichoke and Sprouts Salad (page 120), with The Most Simple Dressing (page 152)

18.

Coconut-Curry Cauliflower (page 216)

Brown Rice (page 172)

19.

Insteada-Tuna Salad Sandwich (page 248)

Enlightenment Smoothie (page 298)

20.

Fried Green Tomatoes (page 214)

Black Beans (page 190)

Brown Rice (page 172)

Lettuce and Tortilla Salad (page 124), with Chimichurri Sauce (page 160)

15.

Wild Nettle Soup (page 57)

Pasta with Pesto (page 98), using angel hair pasta

Simple Steamed Veggies (page 208): kabocha squash

Arugula Salad (page 121)

Sharon's Amazing Chocolate Mousse (page 266)

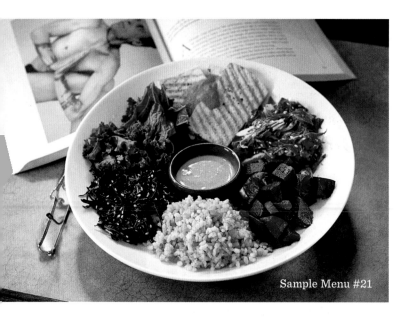

Sample Menu #21

27.

Mashed Potatoes (page 223)

Beans and Faux Chicken (page 196)

Arugula Salad (page 121)

Simple Steamed Veggies (page 208):
corn on the cob, zucchini, and green beans

28.

Maharini Dal (page 61)

Brown Rice Salad (page 125)

Simple Steamed Veggies (page 208): beets

Bankalicious Raw Cacao "Ice Cubes"
(page 290)

29.

Cream of Celery Soup (page 45)

Tempeh Croutons (page 200)

Quinoa with Corn (page 182)

Potato-Zucchini Salad (page 141)

30.

Faux Chicken Pasta (page 110),
minus the pasta

Kasha with Black-Eyed Peas (page 184)

Very Simple Shredded Beet Salad (page 134)

Endive and Walnut Salad (page 119)

Pumpkin Pie (page 285)

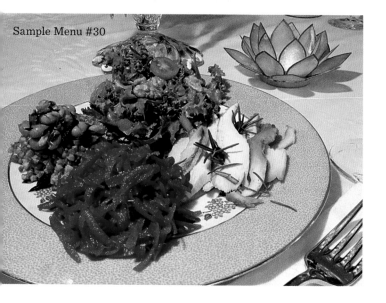

Sample Menu #30

21-Day
Cleansing Diets

Even though a vegan diet is healthier than a meat- or dairy-based diet, sometimes you need a way to boost your immune system, cleanse toxins, reset your metabolism, or even lose a few unwanted pounds. That's the time to go on a cleansing diet. Cleansing through diet is also very powerful when making the transition from meat eater to vegan.

Allow me to share with you two different twenty-one-day cleansing diets. You could call them fasts because they entail restricting your food choices. Once a year I go into retreat and follow one of these diet plans, and have personally received much benefit, and that is why I want to share these diets with you. The first one is the *Bland* diet, and it basically involves eating porridge and a blended salad every day and omitting all salt, spices, oils, and sugars. The second is the *Raw* diet on which you mainly eat salads, smoothies, and juices.

I suggest you pick one of these diets and stay on it for twenty-one days to receive the greatest benefit. If twenty-one days is too much, you can choose to go on the diet for however long you can—even one day on either of these diets would be beneficial to your system.

But why twenty-one days? Many doctors agree that it takes the body about three weeks for the digestive system to rid itself of toxins and to free us of destructive eating habits and biochemical addictions. Eating meat and dairy is addictive. Dr. Neal Barnard explains in his book *Breaking the Food Seduction* that "scientific tests suggest that meat and dairy have subtle drug-like qualities. As meat and dairy touch your tongue, opiates are released in the brain. Also, interestingly enough, meat stimulates a surprisingly strong release of insulin, which is involved in the release of dopamine in the brain, which is the feel-good chemical turned on by every single drug of abuse—opiates, nicotine, cocaine, alcohol, amphetamines, and everything else. Dopamine is what powers the brain's pleasure center. Beef and cheese cause a bigger insulin release than pasta."[25]

Since we all want to be happy and free and to feel good, viewing ourselves with compassion is essential for the success of any diet program. Guilt-tripping and negative projection are never helpful. When we free ourselves from our destructive addictions, we discover that within our own bodies is a complete pharmaceutical laboratory that can generate the well-being we seek without having to look outside of ourselves. But to become independent like that, we must first experience our own bodies when they are not hampered by addiction. This experience reveals the innate intelligence of our bodies, and it is very empowering.

If you feel that going from the SAD (Standard American Diet), consisting mostly of meat and dairy products, to a 100 percent organic, vegan diet overnight may be too much, don't beat yourself up or pressure yourself to change all at once. Instead, try either of these cleansing diets for one day without feeling you have to commit to it or to a vegan diet for the rest of your life, and see what happens. Do it with a sense of adventure. Following either of these cleansing diets will give your digestive organs a rest, as well as gently help your body to transition to a more healthful way of eating. If you can follow one of these diets for the full twenty-one days, you will be able to reset your metabolism and help to free yourself of biochemical addictions triggered by food. And even if you are already vegan, if you drink coffee and tea, and eat sugar and processed soy and wheat gluten products, doing a cleanse can give your system a rest from these taxing foods. After the cleanse, when you start to reincorporate a variety of foods back into your daily meals, you will find that you have an improved appetite, enabling you to better enjoy the taste of food. Your body will greatly appreciate it, as will all of the animals and plants and the greater world we all share.

Both of these cleansing diets are vegan (100 percent plant-based) diets, but they are more restrictive than a "normal" vegan diet. They eliminate many foods that, though vegan, can obstruct the body's ability to maintain optimum health. Nonorganic food, gluten, soy, oil, drugs, alcohol, caffeine, salt, and sugar are abstained from totally or ingested only in small amounts. Why restrict these foods? Wheat, gluten, and soy often cause allergenic reactions. Oil is eliminated (or minimized) to help you lose unwanted weight as well as to give the gallbladder and liver a rest from metabolizing fats. Drugs, alcohol, and caffeine are eliminated to help clear the thinking mind and to help you reflect on the habits you use to deal with stress or to provide a sense of relaxation. Elimination of drugs, alcohol, and caffeine also provides the nervous system and internal organs, especially the adrenals, liver, and kidneys, a rest from having to process these physiologically challenging substances. You will get some naturally occurring salt and sugar found in the foods you will be eating, but no added table salt or sugar is allowed on the diet. Minimizing your salt intake will help to release excess fluids from your cells and reduce puffiness. Many times when we feel we look fat, it is not fat we are seeing but water retention. Eliminating sugar helps to stabilize the overall metabolism so that you will be less prone to cravings and binges. It is important that you do your best to eat only organic food while on a cleansing diet, in order to minimize adding any new toxins into your body.

IMPORTANT NOTE: Neither of these diets will work as a cleansing diet unless you are eliminating sufficiently. You should be having at least one good bowel movement every day. If you become constipated, drink a cup of herbal laxative tea in the morning and/or evening before bed. Enemas can also be used to help maintain a good flushing of the system.

The 21-Day Bland Cleansing Diet

This is by no means a starvation diet. There is ample food with much fiber, so you will not feel hungry and your bowels will most likely have no problem with constipation. Because the food you will be eating will be mostly blended or porridge-like, it will aid in digestion and give your jaw a rest as well. The raw sauerkraut will provide naturally occurring acidophilus to further aid in digestion.

Basically you will be eating oatmeal for breakfast, fresh vegetable juice or raw soup or fruit for lunch, and a porridge-type soup, steamed vegetable, and raw sauerkraut for dinner, with lots of water and herbal teas between meals.

WHAT YOU WILL NEED

Gluten-free oatmeal

Brown rice

Red lentils

Assortment of fresh vegetables for steaming, making juice, and making raw soup

Fresh fruit

Raw sauerkraut

Powdered spirulina

Herbal non-caffeinated tea(s)

Laxative tea (brands like Smooth Move, Get Regular)

Pure water

USEFUL APPLIANCES

Juicer

Food processor and/or blender

THE PLAN FOR THE BLAND DIET

Breakfast

Herbal tea

Oatmeal (made with ½ cup dry, gluten-free oatmeal and water)

Lunch

6 to 12 ounces fresh vegetable juice or a Raw Soup (pages 91–95), but omit the olive oil and salt, or 1 or 2 pieces of fresh fruit

Dinner

8-ounce bowl Kitcheri (page 59), but omit the salt

4 ounces Simple Steamed Veggies (page 208)—your choice, but don't add salt or oil

¼ cup raw sauerkraut—you can make your own (see www.wildfermentation.com) or buy some, but make sure it's raw

SOME TIPS

- Drink lots of water during the day (try adding a squeeze of fresh lemon juice), and drink herbal tea or ginger-lemon tea whenever you want to.
- If you can't go without caffeine, then drink a cup of white, green, oolong, or black tea in the morning. If you can't go without something sweet in your tea, use stevia or a small amount of agave or maple syrup.
- Don't put any sugar, sweeteners, salt, soy sauce, or other spices or condiments on your food.
- Don't use any oil or margarine on your food.
- Don't use any soy milk or other types of milk.
- If you normally take vitamins or other supplements, you may continue to do so, but make sure they are organic and vegan (no gelatin capsules).

The 21-Day Raw Cleansing Diet

This diet is basically a 100 percent raw diet predominately made up of chlorophyll-rich green vegetables, but it can also be modified to include some cooked foods, including steamed vegetables and light soup.

WHAT YOU WILL NEED

Assortment of fresh vegetables and fruits

Ginger

Herbal non-caffeinated tea(s)

Laxative tea (brands like Smooth Move, Get Regular)

Lemons

Powdered spirulina

Powdered vegetable stock or bouillon cubes

Pure water

Sprouts: alfalfa, clover, mung bean, etc.

Breakfast

One cup of herbal tea—chamomile, peppermint, licorice, or ginger-lemon is good. After about 20 minutes, drink a large (10- to 12-ounce) glass of fresh green vegetable juice (not bottled, canned, or processed).

Lunch

Any Raw Soup (pages 91–95), but omit the salt and oil, or 1 or 2 pieces fresh fruit

Dinner

A large salad made with only raw vegetables, dressed with lemon juice and no more than 1 tablespoon olive oil

MODIFICATIONS: Breakfast, lunch, and dinner can be switched. This is a 100 percent raw cleansing diet, but if this diet seems too severe for you, then add one of the following for either lunch or dinner:

- Another large (10- to 12-ounce) glass of fresh green vegetable juice
- Another serving of raw soup, but omit the salt and oil, or 1 or 2 pieces fresh fruit
- ½ to 1 cup Simple Steamed Veggies (page 208)
- 1 cup hot vegetable broth (1 tablespoon powdered vegetable stock or 1 cube of vegetable bouillon dissolved in boiling water)
- If you can't go without caffeine, then drink a cup of white, green, oolong, or black tea in the morning. If you can't go without something sweet in your tea, use stevia or a small amount of agave or maple syrup.

SOME TIPS

- Drink lots of water during the day (try adding a squeeze of fresh lemon juice), and drink herbal tea or ginger-lemon tea whenever you want to.
- Use no more than 2 tablespoons olive oil or flaxseed oil per day, less if you can.
- Limit or eliminate your use of salt.
- Try to go without sweeteners, or limit to stevia or no more than 2 teaspoons a day of agave or maple syrup, no white or brown sugar, even if it's organic.
- Don't use any soy milk or other types of milk.
- If you normally take vitamins or other supplements, you may continue to do so, but make sure they are organic and vegan (no gelatin capsules).

Resources

BOOKS

Animals as Persons, by Gary Francione
Animal Liberation, by Peter Singer
Battered Birds Crated Herds, by Gene Bauston
Becoming Vegan, by Brenda Davis and Vesanto Melina
Breaking the Food Seduction, by Neal Barnard
The China Study, by T. Colin Campbell and Thomas
    M. Campbell II
Crazy Sexy Cancer Tips, by Kris Carr
Crazy Sexy Diet, by Kris Carr
Crazy Sexy Kitchen, by Kris Carr
Diet for a New America, by John Robbins
Dominion, by Matthew Scully
Dr. Neal Barnard's Program for Reversing Diabetes,
    by Neal Barnard
Empty Cages, by Tom Regan
Eternal Treblinka, by Charles Patterson
Farm Sanctuary, by Gene Baur
Flaming Arrows, by Rod Coronado
The Food Revolution, by John Robbins
Free the Animals, by Ingrid Newkirk
From Dusk till Dawn, by Keith Mann
Hope's Edge, by Frances and Anna Moore Lappe
The Inner Art of Vegetarianism, by Carol J. Adams
The Joy of Vegan Baking, by Colleen Patrick-Goudreau
The Mad Cowboy, by Howard Lyman
Making Kind Choices, by Ingrid Newkirk
One Can Make a Difference, by Ingrid Newkirk
101 Reasons Why I'm a Vegetarian, by Pamela Rice
Peace to All Beings, by Judy Carman
Quantum Wellness, by Kathy Freston
Seeds of Deception, by Jeffrey M. Smith
Skinny Bitch, by Rory Freedman and Kim Barnouin
Slaughterhouse, by Gail A. Eisnitz
Spiritual Nutrition, by Gabriel Cousens
Strolling with Our Kin, by Marc Bekoff
Thanking the Monkey, by Karen Dawn
An Unnatural Order, by Jim Mason
Veganist, by Kathy Freston
The World Peace Diet, by Will Tuttle
Yoga and Vegetarianism, by Sharon Gannon
Your Right to Know, by Andrew Kimbrell

VIDEOS

The Animals Film (full-length documentary on animal
    rights narrated by Julie Christie)
*Behind the Mask: The Story of the People Who Risk
    Everything to Save Animals* (documentary about
    animal rights activists)
Bold Native (a feature film that sheds positive focus on
    the ALF [Animal Liberation Front])
Chew on This (a three-minute film showing reasons to
    be a vegetarian, available subtitled in many
    languages)
Earthlings (full-length documentary on animal rights
    narrated by Joaquin Phoenix)
Food Inc. (full-length documentary about the big
    business of food)
The Future of Food (full-length documentary about
    GMOs [genetically modified foods])
Genetic Roulette (full-length documentary about GMOs
    [genetically modified foods])
Glass Walls (short film about why a vegan diet is best
    narrated by Paul McCartney)

DETOX RETREAT CENTERS

Ann Wigmore Institute, Puerto Rico, www
    .annwigmore.org
Hippocrates Health Institute, West Palm Beach,
    Florida, www.hippocratesinst.org
The Tree of Life Rejuvenation Center—Dr. Gabriel
    Cousens, Patagonia, Arizona, www.treeoflife
    centerus.com

HELPFUL WEBSITES

Abolitionist Approach, www.abolitionistapproach.com
Farm Sanctuary, www.farmsanctuary.org
Howard Lyman Factoids and Links, www.madcowboy
    .com
Humane Society of the United States, www.hsus.org
Karen Dawn Media reports, www.dawnwatch.com
PETA, www.peta.org
Physicians Committee for Responsible Medicine,
    www.pcrm.org
Vegan Outreach, www.veganoutreach.org
Warcry Communications, www.voiceofthevoiceless.org

JIVAMUKTEA CAFÉ

The elegant Jivamuktea Café, located adjacent to the
    Jivamukti Yoga School at 841 Broadway, 2nd Floor,
    New York, NY 10003, USA, serves delicious vegan
    meals seven days a week: www.jivamuktiyoga.com.

Acknowledgments

A book like this is a joint effort. I would like to acknowledge some of those special beings who helped to bring this cookbook into manifestation.

First of all, thank you to David Life, who for the past thirty years has been my chief recipe taster, enthusiastic supporter, and creative partner.

Thank you to Gopal (Paul) Steinberg for his meticulous editing of the manuscript over many years, and especially for assisting me every step of the way to getting this book (and all of my other writings) to publication.

Thank you to the photographers, all of whom happen to be vegan: Connie Hansen and Russell Peacock (aka Guzman), who took most of the photographs in this book. I am amazed at not only their artistry, skill, and perfectionism but at how humble and generous they are—never losing their composure, enthusiasm, and joy for every moment. Also to Jessica Sjöö, who took the initial photographs for the book. She is responsible for the zany "Mad Hatter Tea Party" cover shot.

Words are not enough to express my gratitude to the incomparable Kris Carr for her Foreword, friendship, and continued support for this cookbook project. Kris is a living testament to the transformative power of a joyful vegan diet.

Thank you to my beloved friend and teacher Shyamdas for his prayerful insights and for teaching me many ways to make the cooking, offering, and sharing of food with others the most supreme devotional practice.

My appreciation to David Armstrong, Banka Schneider, Julie Kirkpatrick, Kazim Ali, Oscar G. Maccow, Touria Lamtahaf, Joe Sponzo, Rob Frabone, Colleen Patrick-Goudrea, and Gopal Steinberg for graciously sharing recipes and cooking tips with me.

Thank you to my beloved cat companions, Miten, Nicholas, and So-called, and our deer friends that appear in some of the photos taken in Woodstock.

Blessings to Pinar Yigit for traveling to a small village in Turkey to have Sufi hats handmade for David and me and then sending them to us so that we could wear them to the "Mad Hatter Tea Party" depicted on the cover of the book.

Huge thanks, respect, and blessings to the extraordinarily hardworking past and present staff of Jivamuktea Café in New York City. In particular I want to acknowledge David Armstrong, Ayinde Howell, Kevin Archer, Oscar G. Maccow, and Touria Lamtahaf for working alongside me for many years to develop the elegant atmosphere and delicious dishes that are served seven days a week in our café.

Thank you to Radhanath Swami and the devotees at the Radhagopinath Temple in Mumbai, especially Pallika Mataji, Madhurya Lila, and Damodar Prabhu, for helping me test the recipe for the Chocolate Ice Cream Cake.

I am grateful to my friend Rob Frabone for introducing me to George Gilbert, who provided legal advice.

Without the enthusiastic support so graciously given by my incredible editor, Megan Newman, this book would not exist. Also if it hadn't been for Gabriel Heymann and Nancy Baumgarten, I would not have met Megan—so thank you, Gabe and Nancy, for orchestrating that magical meeting. Also special thanks to Gabrielle Campo, Lisa Johnson, and the whole production team at Penguin.

A cookbook photo shoot is a big production involving many people to make sure the shots show the food in the best possible light and arrangement. We had a brilliant team who took the utmost care with every detail: the amazing Travis Manning from Scheimpflug, who assisted the photographic duo Guzman; food stylist Victoria Granof, assisted by Anna Billingskog; April Dechagas and Beth Filla, who tested recipes for me; and Jason McClusky, who washed dishes for days and days—that's a lot of dishes and pots to scrub! And to Ganeshdas Menjivar and Linda Zhang, who stand as pillars of support for all my projects.

And to all the kind people who have committed to eating a vegan diet—thank you for daring to care about the happiness, well-being, and liberation of other animals—blessings to you!

Notes

1 For a fuller discussion of this point, see Sharon Gannon, *Yoga and Vegetarianism: The Diet of Enlightenment* (San Rafael, CA: Mandala, 2008), 71–74.

2 See http://farmusa.org/statistics11.html.

3 See http://www.who.int/water_sanitation_health/mdg1/en/.

4 See http://www.peta.org/issues/animals-used-for-food/meat-wastes-natural-resources.aspx.

5 Ibid.

6 John Robbins, *Diet for a New America* (Tiburon, CA: HJ Kramer, 1998), 367.

7 See http://www.fao.org/ag/magazine/0612sp1.htm.

8 John Robbins, *The Food Revolution* (Berkeley, CA: Conari Press, 2001), 19.

9 World Cancer Research Fund and American Institute for Cancer Research, *Food, Nutrition, and the Prevention of Cancer* (Washington, DC: World Cancer Research Fund/American Institute for Cancer Research, 1997), 456–57.

10 See http://www.pcrm.org/health/diabetes-resources/diabetes-success-stories.

11 See http://prime.peta.org/2012/11/longer.

12 Maria Esposito, "Is High Cholesterol Harming Your Sex Life?" Fox News, August 13, 2008, <http://www.foxnews.com/story/0,2933,403384,00.html>; see also http://www.peta.org/living/vegetarian-living/impotence.aspx.

13 See http://www.vrg.org/nutrition/iron.php.

14 See http://www.nutritionmd.org/health_care_providers/hematology/ironanemia_nutrition.html.

15 See http://www.pcrm.org/health/health-topics/calcium-and-strong-bones.

16 See http://www.vibrancyuk.com/dairy.html.

17 See http://www.diseaseproof.com/archives/osteoporosis-choose-vegetable-calcium-over-animal-calcium.html.

18 Paul Watson, "Consider the Fishes," *VegNews,* March–April 2003, 27.

19 See http://www.downtoearth.org/health/general-health/steps-to-end-world-hunger.

20 Marc Bekoff, *Strolling with Our Kin* (New York: Lantern Books, 2000), 70.

21 See *Behind the Mask: The Story of the People Who Risk Everything to Save Animals,* directed by Shannon Keith (Valley Village, CA: Uncaged Films, 2006), DVD.

22 R. Mazess, "Bone Mineral Content of North Alaskan Eskimos," *American Journal of Clinical Nutrition* 9 (1974): 916–25.

23 Geoff Bond, *Deadly Harvest: The Intimate Relationship Between Our Health and Our Food* (Garden City Park, NY: Square One Publishers, 2007), 91.

24 See http://www.chiro.org/nutrition/FULL/Defeating_Free_Radicals.shtml and http://www.drweil.com/drw/u/id/QAA358078.

25 Neal Barnard, *Breaking the Food Seduction* (New York: St. Martin's Press, 2004), 63–64.

Index